AF289849

Schriftenreihe Neurologie — Neurology Series

16

Rainer Heene

Experimental Myopathies and Muscular Dystrophy

*Studies in the Formal Pathogenesis of the Myopathy of
2,4-Dichlorophenoxyacetate*

With 17 Figures

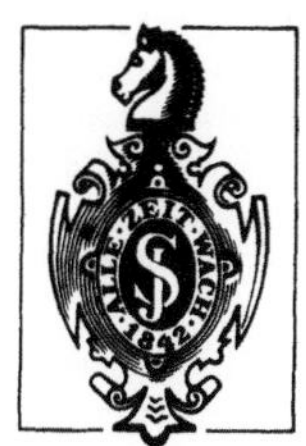

Springer-Verlag Berlin · Heidelberg · New York 1975

Prof. Dr. med. RAINER HEENE
Oberarzt an der Universitäts-Nervenklinik
3550 Marburg/Lahn, Ortenbergstraße 8

ISBN-13:978-3-642-66202-7   e-ISBN-13:978-3-642-66200-3
DOI: 10.1007/978-3-642-66200-3

Library of Congress Cataloging in Publication Data. Heene, Rainer, 1930— Experimental myopathies and muscular dystrophy (Neurology series; 16). Includes bibliographical references and index. 1. Muscle—Diseases. 2. Pathology, Experimental. 3. Dichlorophenoxyacetic acid—Toxicology. 4. Muscular dystrophy. I. Title. II. Series: Schriftenreihe Neurologie; 16. [DNLM: 1. Muscular diseases—Etiology. 2. Muscular dystrophy—Etiology. 3. 0,2,4-D—Toxicity. W1 SC344 Bd. 16 / WE550 H458e] RC925.5.H43 616.7'4'07 75-20180

Contents

Indroduction

In attempts to understand the pathogenesis of primary myopathies
in man, the study of experimental myopathies in warm-blooded animals is of fundamental interest. Among these, the hereditary myopathies of the mouse and of the chicken and the myopathy induced
by vitamin-E deficiency are particularly important, as well as
the myopathies that follow treatment with corticosteroids or
chloroquine. Morphological and physiological studies of these
model diseases in animals are essential, less with regard to the
etiology than to the formal pathogenesis of muscle diseases.
This means that the findings must be considered as relatively
nonspecific. The specific etiology of the various primary myopathies in man and in animals involves problems of molecular
biology, which at present are still largely unsolved. It thus
falls within the scope of formal pathogenesis to trace the symptoms back as closely as possible to the hypothetical primary
lesion. Such an attempt has been undertaken in the present study,
which refers essentially to the earliest alterations in skeletal
muscle, as detected by histochemical and histological methods.
It was established by the studies of RANVIER (1874, cited by
(262)) that "red" skeletal muscle differs from "white" with regard, for instance, to speed of contraction, which is higher in
white than in red muscle. Following RANVIER's observations, the
different types of muscle fibre can now be characterized by a
variety of biochemical, morphological, and physiological para-
meters. When all these findings are taken into account, the
important question for the formal pathogenesis of primary myopathies is whether one or the other type of muscle fibres is predilectively involved. The histochemical differentiation of fibre
types in skeletal muscle thus constitutes an essential prerequi-
site of myopathology. Statements concerning the primary involvement of one fibre type in the advanced stages of myopathy are
of limited value because of the secondary changes that occur in
fibres which are not predilectively involved in the disease.
This applies in particular to the hereditary myopathies, in which
an inborn defect may already become apparent at the fetal stages
of differentiation of the fibre types of skeletal muscle. Since
biopsies can be performed only at rather late stages of human
muscle development, specifity of fibre type in the earliest
alterations can hardly be ascertained. Thus, apart from the hereditary myopathies, our interest is drawn to those varieties of
muscular disease in which controlled lesions can supply information concerning the predilective involvement of red or white
fibres in the myopathic process.

The myopathy induced by injections of 2,4-dichlorophenoxyacetate
(2,4-D), a common herbicide, provides a good example. The present

study deals with our histological and histochemical findings relating to this myopathy in the white rat. The earliest alterations in skeletal muscle were studied with particular care and as a result it proved necessary to revise some earlier findings (138, 141) concerning the sequelae of the acute intoxication of rats with 2,4-D. Further, it was possible to give a more conclusive interpretation of the histochemical effects of 2,4-D in vitro on muscle phosphorylase (139). For this purpose gelatin film incubation methods had to be newly designed. Following the discussion of the findings, the myopathy induced by 2,4-D is compared with other experimental myopathies and its significance examined in relation to the problems of progressive muscular dystrophy in man. The true etiology of the disease, i.e. the primary metabolic action of 2,4-D in the muscle fibre, is a biochemical problem, the solution of which necessarily exceeds the scope of this pathogenetic study.

From several points of view it seemed important to perform equivalent studies on the heart and on the liver. Histochemically, the myocardium of the ventricles is a red muscle which, in case of predilective involvement of one or the other type of fibres in the skeletal muscle, should either be susceptible to the myopathic process or unaffected by it. Thus, the involvement of the heart early in the disease would be crucial for our evaluation of which type of fibres in skeletal muscle is predilectively altered.

Liver and skeletal muscle are tightly linked in glycogen metabolism. Thus the hepatotoxic effects of 2,4-D cannot be strictly distinguished from the hypothetical changes induced in the liver by the myopathic process. Nevertheless, it seems reasonable to consider this problem in the light of specific reports on alterations in liver function in primary myopathies of man (145).

The account of the effects of 2,4-D is preceded by a review of findings in various experimental myopathies in animals. Here too, special attention has been paid to the aspects of predilective fibre involvement in skeletal muscle and to alterations of the heart muscle.

Experimental Myopathies

A. Pharmacotoxic Myopathies

I. Myopathy of Corticosteroids

In a light-microscopic study of the myopathy induced by corticosteroid treatment, ELLIS (92, 93) described an early segmental swelling of the muscle fibres accompanied by varying degrees of eosinophilia of the sarcoplasm. Since histochemical techniques were not used, predilective involvement of one or the other type of muscle fibres could not be demonstrated. Even under prolonged treatment, when severe changes were present in skeletal muscle, the myocardium appeared to be unchanged. Infiltration with fat and focal necrosis were found in the liver. The alterations in skeletal muscle were those of a primary myopathy and were fully reversed when treatment was discontinued.

With the electron microscope (3) an accumulation of glycogen in the subsarcolemmal space was observed at an early stage in the disease process. Myofibrillar structure was unimpaired. More advanced stages could be characterized by a decrease in glycogen content prior to typical necrosis of the muscle fibre. In an intermediate phase of the process, reversible swelling and disintegration of mitochondrial cristae as well as dissociation of the Z line and swelling of components of the sarcoplasmic reticulum were demonstrated (237). Only at advanced stages of fibre necrosis, including phagocytosis, could regenerative signs be observed. These were inconspicuous as long as treatment was continued. The alterations in the diaphragm of rabbits given corticosteroids indicated predilective involvement of granular red muscle fibres (67, 68). Glycogen accumulation was seen in both types of muscle fibre. Necrosis was preceded by swelling of the fibres and by proliferation of the sarcoplasmic reticulum. Lipid deposits increased, especially in red fibres.

In a comparative morphological study of the effects of cortisone acetate and of fluorocorticosteroids (triamcinolone) on muscle, SMITH (275) demonstrated particularly high myotoxic activities of the fluorinated compound. An increase in glycogen content and a decrease in phosphorylase activity in the muscle fibres preceded the onset of histological change. This was paralleled by increased activity of the oxidative enzymes in white muscle fibres, which presented a coarse intermyofibrillar pattern. White muscle fibres were predilectively prone to myopathic changes, i.e. to initial swelling. The myocardium was unaltered. SMITH concluded that one of the basic effects of triamcinolone on the muscle cell could be suppression of the activation of phosphorylase, accompanied by increased yields in oxidative metabolism. A decrease in the activity of muscle phosphorylase effected by corticosteroids was confirmed by biochemical methods (175, 301). This effect is dose-dependent and can be antagonized by epinephrine (175). Biochemical studies on rats (238) given intraperitoneal injections of triamcinolone revealed loss of glycogen from the muscle cell within 4 hours, and an increase in glycogen content at 8 to 12 h following injection. VIGNOS and GREENE (302) were able to demonstrate that the severity of the muscular changes in the rabbit was dependent on the proportion of white type-2 fibres present in any of the sampled muscles. Contrary to red muscle, the respiratory rate of white muscle was shown to be diminished in these experiments.

As viewed with the electron microscope, an early stage, which can be characterized by proliferation of mitochondria, especially in white muscle fibres (295, 296), is seen to be followed by a decrease in the number of these organelles in both red and white muscle fibres. Myofibrillar alterations occurred in particular in red muscle. Changes which were observed in the lateral vastus muscle of rats 2 h after a single injection of 20 mg/kg of triamcinolone acetonide included mitochondrial proliferation in the subsarcolemmal zone and loss of mitochondria from the central parts of the white muscle fibres (49). In man, symptomatic myopathies were seen to develop following therapeutic injections of fluorinated corticosteroids (2). The alterations of skeletal muscle in these conditions resembled those in the experimental animals. Different degrees of muscular involvement in the human cases were explained by assuming that the biopsies had been performed at different intervals during the biphasic mitochondrial reaction mentioned above. In man, extensive subsarcolemmal accumulations of glycogen were also observed. From these findings, some of which are still contradictory, it can be concluded that in the early stages of corticosteroid myopathies white muscle fibres will be predilectively altered (275). Differences in the muscular involvement may result from differences in the myotoxicity of the various compounds, of which triamcinolone is the most effective. This substance, however, did not induce cardiac alterations (92).

II.   Myopathy of Chloroquine

Predilective damage to red muscle fibres was observed in the myopathy following injection of chloroquine (81, 219). In the rabbit, weakness and atrophy of skeletal muscle were far less marked than the severe cardiomyopathic changes. Vacuolar degeneration and necrosis of heart muscle fibres were observed together with histiocytic reaction (4, 32, 277, 303). In skeletal muscle only single-fibre necrosis could be demonstrated. White muscle fibres appeared unchanged and their histochemical phosphorylase and ATPase reactions were intact (4, 277).

In an electron-microscopic study of the red soleus and the white gastrocnemius muscle of rats (192), the soleus muscle was found to be more seriously involved than the gastrocnemius at any stage of the disease. Formation of so-called myelin bodies and of vacuoles with double membranes as well as longitudinal division of muscle fibres was described. MACDONALD and ENGEL (192) concluded from their comprehensive morphological and biochemical findings that chloroquine would act primarily by stimulating the formation of phospholipid membranes from the longitudinal and transverse tubular system of the muscle fibre. Electromyographic recordings in man (222) indicate that chloroquine exerts myo- and neurotoxic effects.

Plasmocid, a compound of quinoline, exceeds chloroquine in its myotoxic action (146). Injection of this substance gave rise in the myocardium to swelling and aggregation of mitochondria whose internal structure had disintegrated (66). Correspondingly, the histochemical activities of succinodehydrogenase and of cytochromeoxydase were reduced or were entirely absent (19, 303). Following the injection of small amounts (12 mg/kg) of this substance, selective damage to actin filaments and Z bands were observed as well as swelling of the sarcoplasmic reticulum (243).

III. Myotonia-Myopathy Syndrome of 20,25-Diazacholesterol

Only a few studies have been concerned with the question of predilective involvement of muscle fibres in the myotonia-myopathy syndrome of 20,25-diazacholesteroldihydrochloride (278, 314).

Using electrophysiological methods, GOODGOLD and EBERSTEIN (125) demonstrated that in rats treated with 25-azacholesterol the myotonic reaction developed earlier in white than in red muscle (83, 125). Male animals were more prone to myotonia than females. Since the myotonic reaction could not be abolished by curare nor by section of the sciatic nerve, it was concluded that 25-aza-cholesterol acted upon the membrane of the muscle fibre. This was recently established biochemically by findings of SEILER et al. (267). The formation of vacuoles in degenerating muscle fibres under prolonged treatment with 20,25-diazacholesterol (313) could be shown to result from dilatations of the transverse tubular system (265).

IV. Myopathy of Vincristine

In a comprehensive morphological and biochemical study of the myopathy following acute intoxication of rats with vincristine, CLARKE et al. (56) described marked differences in the involvement of different muscles in the disease process. The gastrocnemius muscle displayed only minor changes and the soleus muscle was completely spared. Conversely, different degrees of involvement of type-2 fibres were observed in the brachial biceps muscle. Under the light microscope the minimal alterations presented as a coarse basophilic granular structure in the sarcoplasm. This alteration could be assessed by means of the electron microscope as due to swelling of the mitochondria and to the formation of membranous lipid layers, known as myelin bodies. Focal disintegration of the intermyofibrillar network could be observed in more advanced stages of the disease process. At terminal stages of muscular alteration, fibre necrosis was accompanied by loss of histochemical reactivity for glycogen and for phosphorylase. Eleven days after treatment had been discontinued reversal of these changes was apparent. Histochemically, defects of intermyofibrillar structure could be demonstrated at this time. The authors concluded that changes in the intermyofibrillar structures, i.e. in the sarcoplasmic reticulum and in mitochondria, would precede necrosis of muscle fibres. The corresponding ultrastructural alterations were demonstrated by BRADLEY (33) in the guinea pig subjected to acute or chronic intoxication with vincristine. He showed that in this species the neuroaxonal changes, i.e. vacuolization of the axoplasm preceding neuroaxonal degeneration, were not an outstanding feature of this neuromyopathy. An extensive morphological similarity can be shown to exist between the myopathy of vincristine on the one hand and that of 2,4-D on the other.

B.   The Myopathy of Vitamin-E Deficiency

The myopathy of vitamin-E deficiency develops in different species of warm-blooded animals after widely differing periods of continuous avitaminosis (91, 102, 223, 246, 311). Myopathy is only one manifestation of this condition. Thus EINARSON and RINGSTED (91) could already demonstrate, besides myopathic changes, alterations in the dorsal columns, in the pyramidal tracts and in the anterior horn cells of the spinal cord of the rat. These authors stated that vitamin-E deficiency gives rise to both myopathic and neurological lesions. WOLF and PAPPENHEIMER (315) suggested that the alterations in the anterior horn cells were unlikely to be due to vitamin-E deficiency. More recently, presynaptic axonal swelling in the nuclei of the dorsal column was found in vitamin-E deficient rats (117). These findings, like those in the neuromyopathy of vincristine, indicate that in "primary" myopathies the possibility of an involvement of organs other than the skeletal muscle should always be considered.

ANGELINI et al. (8) found that the level of M isozymes of lactate dehydrogenase in the serum of vitamin-E deficient rabbits was lowered both absolutely and in relation to the level of H isozymes. As the latter are characteristic of red skeletal muscle and of heart muscle, the authors' findings could be consistent with predilective involvement of white muscle fibres in the disease. Parallel experiments showed increased activities of creatine phosphate kinase and of aldolase in the serum (7). Histological alterations were prominent in the white adductor magnus as compared to the red soleus muscle. Contrary to findings in the rat, involvement of the liver could not be demonstrated in the rabbit (7, 8, 50, 318). Disseminated fibre necrosis, hyaline degeneration, central rowing of nuclei as a regenerative sign, and increased basophilia of the sarcoplasm could be observed in the affected animals. The suckling rat proved most sensitive to vitamin-E deficiency. There was evidence of involvement of other organs in addition to muscle, and in particular of the central nervous system (191).

PAPPENHEIMER, considering the effect of muscular activity on the outcome of myopathic lesions, demonstrated, that the development of changes in the gastrocnemius muscle could be slowed down by severance of the Achilles tendon (227) or the sciatic nerve. The latter measure had this effect only when performed between the 5th and the 17th day of life (228).

Predilective involvement of white muscle fibres has also been described in vitamin-E deficient chickens (190, 220). Glycogen content and phosphorylase activity of the muscle decreased early in this condition. The relation of active to total phosphorylase, as opposed to findings in the experimental atrophy of denervation, remained constant (190). Involvement of heart muscle could not be observed in the rabbit but was present in the mouse, sheep and calf (299). In all cases the cardiac lesions were less marked than those of the skeletal muscle (194, 196). The invasion of altered cardiac muscle fibres by macrophages was inconspicuous. Necrotic fibres were predominantly replaced by connective tissue. Purkinje fibres were on the whole unaffected by the process.

The earliest changes that could be observed with the electron microscope in skeletal muscle of diseased rabbits consisted of mitochondrial swelling (299) and destruction of the cristae. Alterations of the Z line and vacuolar degeneration of myofibrils (258) prior to disintegration of the sarcomere structure were also described. Loss of anisotropia of the sarcomere in the disease process was hypothetically related to loss of the specific contractile protein actomyosin (6). The activities of lysosomal enzymes increased in parallel with the severity of the myopathic changes in white skeletal muscle (50, 318). The ineffectiveness of treatment with vitamin E in mice with hereditary dystrophy as well as in muscular dystrophy of man (108) seems to show that different metabolic mechanisms are involved in the hereditary dystrophies on the one hand and vitamin-E deficiency on the other. This suggestion was confirmed by the finding that the level of tocopherol in the muscle and other organs of patients with muscular dystrophy was within normal limits (195).

It is, however, remarkable that SCHOLLER et al., treating dystrophic mice with coenzyme Q_7, which is chemically related to vitamin E, succeeded in prolonging the lifespan of the animals from 8 to 10 months and in effecting a transient improvement in the myopathic symptoms (263).

The specific action of vitamin E on the metabolism is still unknown. Its hydroquinone compound, related in structure to coenzyme Q_{10} (113, 186), can inhibit the oxidation of lipids in vivo (318). The development of a myopathy of vitamin-E deficiency can be prevented by supplying selenium to the animals in their food (103, 166, 266).

The Rottnest quokka (Setonix brachyurus) is subject to a spontaneously occurring myopathy of vitamin-E deficiency. In their natural biotope, an island off the southwest coast of Australia, these animals are already exposed to a situation of relative vitamin-E deficiency (170). This condition becomes critical when the animals are kept deficient in vitamin E for experimental purposes over longer periods. A severe myopathy then develops (171), which includes involvement of the heart (80). Nutritional supply of vitamin E to the animals exerts therapeutic and prophylactic effects.

C. Hereditary Myopathies in Animals

Among the hereditary myopathies in warm-blooded animals, the muscular dystrophies of the chicken (13, 169), of the white mouse (strain dydy129 (133, 210)) and of the Syrian hamster (168) have been most thoroughly studied.

I. Muscular Dystrophy of the Chicken

HOLLIDAY et al. (149) showed that in muscular dystrophy of the chicken hypertrophy of the white muscle is prominent during the first weeks of life, followed by atrophy, with replacement of muscle tissue by fat. Histochemically, predilective involvement of white muscle fibres could be established (14, 169, 297). The alterations to the muscle resembled those of vitamin-E deficiency in this species. As to the usual histological criteria of myopathies, it must be mentioned that in the normal chicken the nuclei of white muscle fibres are not typically situated in a subsarcolemmal position, but can be seen scattered over the whole square section of the fibres. Hypertrophied and partly vacuolated muscle fibres were found to be characteristic of the changes in the white breast muscle of the dystrophic chicken. Histochemically, increased activities of oxidative enzymes were observed, comparable to those seen in normal red muscle fibres and in the early developmental stages of the muscle fibre (64, 297). In the electron microscope the vacuoles were shown to arise from distensions of the sarcoplasmic reticulum into which sarcoplasm was incorporated, possibly by way of pinocytosis (54). The great pectoral muscle of the normal chicken changes during development from red muscle at hatching to white muscle in the adult animal (63). Histochemically this change is paralleled by an increase in the activity of phosphorylase and by a decrease in the activity of succinodehydrogenase (62, 63, 64, 65). Dystrophic animals fail to display these developmental changes. The original activity ratios of the two enzymes persist from the time of hatching. From these findings it was concluded that phosphorylase activity would be a limiting factor in the development of the activities of other glyco-

lytic enzymes (63). ASHMORE and DOERR (11), in a biochemical
study, reached different conclusions. Prior to the onset of
degenerative histological alterations, the authors found clearly increased phosphorylase activities in both the red adductor
muscle, which was spared from dystrophic changes, and the white
pectoral muscle. It was only with advanced myopathic changes
that the activity of phosphorylase fell below normal. The
authors supposed that differences between their own and COSMOS'
(63) findings might be explained by different breeding conditions. As stated by ASHMORE and DOERR (12) in a comparative
histochemical study, the period of differentiation of A (α-
white) from the ontogenetically preceding C (α-red) fibres in
the chicken must be regarded as a critical step in which the
myopathic condition becomes manifest. In accordance with the
hypothesis that the maturation of white muscle fibres is disturbed in the disease, the level of H isozymes of lactate dehydrogenase characteristic of red muscle was found to be increased in dystrophic muscle (173). Furthermore, in comparative
biochemical and histochemical studies on dystrophic chickens,
highly pronounced alterations of the activities of $NADH_2$-shut-
tle enzymes (α-glycerophosphate dehydrogenase) were found to
occur in the white pectoral muscle, whereas the caudal tibial
muscle of these animals, comprising a larger proportion of red
fibres, was unaffected (236).

With electrophysiological methods, a decrease in spontaneous
transmitter release at the presynaptic membrane, an increased
duration of the end-plate potential, and alterations at the
post-synaptic membrane with changes in the refractory period
following stimulation of the nerve were reported from studies
in the latissimus dorsi muscle of dystrophic chickens. These
alterations were interpreted as pointing to an involvement of
the preterminal motor innervation in the disease process. It
was suggested that a failure in the neurotrophic regulation of
ion fluxes in excitable membranes could bring about the experimental changes (5).

II. Muscular Dystrophy of the Mouse

PEARCE and WALTON (231) compared the histological findings in
the hereditary muscular dystrophy of the mouse with their own
findings in 69 cases of progressive muscular dystrophy and myotonic dystrophy in man. They concluded that from the histological
viewpoint, while the disease in the mouse was related to Duchenne
muscular dystrophy as regards basophilia of the sarcoplasm (206,
232) and the signs of regeneration, it also resembled myotonic
dystrophy. No direct analogy should be drawn between the diseases
in mouse and in man. From biochemical findings on the activity
of creatine kinase in the breast muscle of the dystrophic chick-
en, it was concluded that findings established in one species
cannot be applied without restrictions to another (256). It was
claimed, from the histochemically observed increase in fat content and oxidative enzyme activities in the red muscle fibres of
dystrophic mice, that this fibre type would be predilectively
involved (162, 286). However, the histochemical methods used in

these studies did not provide a reliable distinction of fibre types in dystrophic muscle. In addition, one study (286) was concerned with advanced stages of the disease in which involvement of red muscle fibres as a secondary phenomenon must in fact be expected. FAHIMI and ROY (107), using the histochemical reaction for lactate dehydrogenase with the aid of phenazine-methosulfate (PMS), showed evidence that in the rectus and vastus lateralis muscles of 5-week-old dystrophic mice the primary lesion occurs in white muscle fibres. The earliest changes during fetal life could be determined to the 19th and 20th days of gestation (205); these involved "tertiary" fibres, which in normal animals are phosphorylase-rich precursors of the white fibres.

The succeeding developmental stages in diseased animals displayed multifocal alterations of muscle fibres with concomitant loss of phosphorylase activity from the tertiary fibres. Fibre atrophy was constantly associated with loss of phosphorylase activity. Red muscle fibres appeared unchanged. With the reaction for lactate dehydrogenase the myophatic alterations were manifested as a coarse granular structure of the intermyofibrillar pattern. In a comparative study on the developmental changes of skeletal muscle during the ontogenesis of normal and dystrophic mice (252, 253), the disease process could be characterized as finally resulting in a reduction in the number of muscle fibres. The red soleus muscle was spared from the myopathic process.

Biochemically, in the early stages of murine muscular dystrophy, as in muscular dystrophy of man (74), decreased activities of muscle phosphorylase were found. LEONARD was able to show (189) that whereas the activities of both active and total phosphorylase were decreased in different muscles of dystrophic mice, the ratio between them remained constant. The glycogen content of the muscle was significantly increased in the initial stages of the disease process. By repetitive electrical stimulation of the anterior tibial muscle, a relative increase in active phosphorylase could be induced, exceeding that of controls (257). In dystrophic animals 7 to 8 weeks of age, the total activity of phosphorylase of this muscle was only 75% of that in controls (294). In addition, an unspecific increase in ATPase activity could be demonstrated in the diseased animals. In the gastrocnemius muscle of female animals, at 7 weeks of age, the decrease in the activities of glycolytic enzymes was found to be significantly greater than in the muscle of male littermates (280).

HOOTON and WATTS (154) were the first to give evidence of a possible biochemical defect in the dystrophy of the mouse. They isolated from dystrophic muscle a variety of creatine kinase yielding only half of the activity of the normal enzyme. Studies of the structure of the defective enzyme revealed that it possessed only half the reactive thiol groups of that in controls. An autosomal-recessive mode of inheritance of the enzyme defect was demonstrated. HOOTON and WATTS' findings could not be confirmed in the dystrophy of the chicken (256) or in muscular dystrophy in man (160).

Electrophysiological studies, too, showed evidence of predilective alterations in white muscle fibres. In the gastrocnemius muscle of dystrophic mice a myotonic reaction could be elicited, relaxation being delayed by a factor of 3 (41, 260). Tension output was found to be diminished during both single and tetanic contraction. As opposed to this, relaxation of the soleus muscle was unchanged. Relative loss of weight of this muscle in dystrophic animals was only half of that of the gastrocnemius (41). It was concluded from observations in dystrophic mouse muscle subjected in vitro to different conditions of ionic environment that alterations are brought about by the dystrophic process at calcium-affine sites of the muscle fibre membrane (39, 40, 42). The fatigability of dystrophic white muscle subjected to tetanic stimulation was found to be decreased (59, 148). HARRIS (134) could demonstrate in the predominantly white extensor digitorum longus muscle a decrease in resting potential which was twice that in the red soleus muscle. He pointed out that fast and slowly contracting muscle fibres could be differently involved by the dystrophic process. Earlier studies had not revealed significant decreases in the resting potential of still excitable muscle fibres (58, 200). A slight but significant decrease could be displayed in the gastrocnemius muscle, if the measurements included fibres that had lost their excitability (58, 188). Excitability of intact fibres was increased, giving rise to spontaneous discharges with shortening of the refractory period (58, 188, 200). Spontaneous end-plate activity was similar to that of denervation (60). Experiments on nerve-muscle preparations in dystrophic animals (18, 60) provided evidence of alterations of cholinergic mechanisms. The amount of disposable cholinesterase was markedly decreased, suggesting an increased activity of acetylcholine at the motor end-plate of dystrophic muscle fibres (120). Histochemical studies with the acetyl-thiocholine method in advanced stages of the disease revealed secondary changes in subneural structures (133). These findings indicate that the motor end-plate is also involved in muscular dystrophy of the mouse. Furthermore, it has been shown in electrophysiological studies that the number of motor units in the gastrocnemius and tibialis anterior muscles of dystrophic mice is reduced and that, from the histological point of view, the myelinated intramuscular nerve fibres are decreased in number (135). It has been concluded from these findings that denervation might play a primary role in muscular dystrophy of the mouse. It must be mentioned that loss of neurotrophic function has been claimed to be an essential factor in the pathogenesis of muscular dystrophy in the chicken as well (5). On the ultrastructural level, distension of the sarcoplasmic reticulum and of the mitochondria together with proliferation of the cristae were observed as the earliest changes in the anterior tibial muscle at preclinical stages of the disease in the mouse (240, 241, 312). SHAFIQ et al. (269) found an increase in the number of mitochondria in the soleus and extensor digitorum longus muscles of mice at 2 to 4 months of age, and this increase was still more outstanding in the gastrocnemius muscle. Later in the disease, destruction of myofilaments occurred with dissolution of sarcomere structure and the number and size of intracellular fat droplets increased (22, 241). Focal proliferation of fibres of the embryonic type could be observed (22). The sarcolemmal structure

appeared to be altered when only minute changes in the fibre
structure were present. A sarcolemmal membrane could not be
observed in fibres regenerating in an embryonic fashion (241).
Longitudinal division, as observed in diseased fibres, was
thought to be due to incomplete apposition of neighbouring
fibres (21, 34). Histochemical enzyme activities in these cells
were at a lower level. In any of the regenerating fibres a
prominent Golgi complex could be demonstrated in a subsarcolemmal position (21). Formation of rough endoplasmic reticulum
was observed (307) in the perikaryon of internal nuclei. This
activation of the sarcoplasm (308) was regarded as paralleling
regeneration on the ultrastructural level.

Histologically, the myopathic alterations could be traced back
to embryonic stages of development. In animals that were later
manifestly diseased regenerative phenomena could be observed
in muscle from the 2nd day of postnatal life. Clear histological
changes could be detected at 12 days of life in the tongue and
in muscles of the hind legs, where they presented as coagulation
necrosis and as symptoms suggestive of regeneration (206). Alterations of the tongue were listed as atypical inasmuch as they
formed foci of vacuolar degeneration of the muscle fibres situated symmetrically along the nervous-vascular supply path. The
same histological changes were seen in less prominent form in
heterozygotes that displayed no clinical manifestations of the
disease (206).

Regeneration following mechanical crushing of the gastrocnemius
muscle will proceed faster in dystrophic mice than in controls
(287). Yet there is no differentiation of white muscle fibres;
regeneration does not proceed beyond an earlier stage where a
type of red fibres is formed. Consistent with this, spontaneous
dedifferentiation, yielding a type of red muscle fibres, could
be demonstrated in the course of the disease. These experiments
provide evidence that the dystrophic process can be symptomati-
cally modified by experimental lesions. As demonstrated by
BANKER and DENNY-BROWN (23), this also holds true for denervation of dystrophic muscle.

In contrast to the severe involvement of skeletal muscle, the
myocardium of dystrophic mice was found to be only slightly
changed or completely unaffected by the myopathic process (164,
206, 312). Consistent with this, in muscular dystrophy of the
mouse the potassium concentration in the myocardium was found
to be normal, whereas it was decreased in skeletal muscle (317).

In 5 out of 9 dystrophic mice FORBES and SPERELAKIS (114) described ultrastructural lesions in some of the fibres of the
ventricular myocardium. These alterations consisted in severe
contraction of the myofibrils, together with separation of the
membranes of the intercalated disks with or without disruption
of the desmosomes and of the gap junctions. A marked increase
in the number of the mitochondria could be observed. The range
of size of these organelles was augmented and their cristae
were reduced in number. The longitudinal and transverse tubular
systems appeared to be enlarged. The atrial muscle cells were
not affected. MONCKTON and MARUSYK (214) observed an increase

in the number of nuclei and in the mitochondrial percentage area
of the myocardial cells. Contrary to former findings in dystrophic skeletal muscle (213), the uptake of ^{3}H-leucine and ^{3}H-uri-
dine by the ventricular myocardium was significantly reduced, indicating a decreased synthetic activity of this tissue. As em-
phasized by the authors, these changes suggest atrophy rather
than dystrophy of the myocardium as the underlying process.

The interpretation of the observed increase in enzyme activities
of the pentose phosphate cycle in dystrophic mouse muscle is to
some degree inconclusive. Biochemically, the various enzyme activities were found to be increased in early stages of the disease
(52, 198, 199), but similar changes could also be seen in normal
muscle following denervation (53, 119, 199). In denervated soleus
and gastrocnemius muscle of the rabbit the increase, and in particular that of the activity of glucose-6-phosphate dehydrogenase,
developed in parallel with the amount of collagen in the muscle.
In muscular dystrophy, on the other hand, the increase in the
activities of these enzymes reached a maximum when there was
macrophage invasion of the tissue, and this increased activity
could be related in dystrophy as well to the proliferation of
connective tissue and to the increase in the lipid content of
the muscle (119, 199). These results correspond to similar
findings in progressive muscular dystrophy of man (145).

Histochemically, the increase in activity of glucose-6-phosphate
dehydrogenase, not in the interstitial tissue but in the muscle
fibres themselves, was argued to be one of the earliest signs
of muscle involvement in the disease of the mouse (111, 286, 312).
The skeletal muscle of fetal rhesus monkeys, still a red type
of muscle, biochemically yields high activities of glucose-6-
phosphate dehydrogenase, which decline during ontogenesis (28).
Given the suggestion that the dystrophic process can be characterized as effecting a dedifferentiation of white muscle towards
a type of fetal red muscle (269), the findings in the monkey
would be consistent with the above-mentioned histochemical
changes, which indicate that the increase in pentose-cycle enzymes is brought about in the actual muscle fibre.

III. Muscular Dystrophy of the Hamster

In a thorough study comparing normal hamsters and <u>hamster with
muscular dystrophy</u>, JOHNSON and PEARSE (168) elucidated the
problem of predilective involvement of one fibre type. Red type-
1 fibres of the quadriceps muscle of dystrophic animals displayed greater variability of diameter in particular from the
60th day of life onward. White type-2 fibres were far more severely affected; from the 20th day onwards they showed prominent signs
of atrophy with drastically reduced phosphorylase activity. Later
on, the mean diameter of white fibres approached normal and then
actually exceeded it, accompanied by a large increase in sample
variance. An increasing proportion of type-2 fibres was grossly
hypertrophied, these fibres retaining high levels of phosphorylase activity. Type-3 fibres (corresponding to ATPase 2B fibres
of BROOKE and KAISER (38)) showed less deviation from normal than

type 2 but were more severely affected than type 1. The authors concluded that the level of glycolytic activity - as represented by the histochemical phosphorylase reaction - might be of importance in determining the upper limits of growth in individual muscle fibres, as regards both normal development and hypertrophy of the muscle fibre in response to a myopathic process. It appeared that most of the enzyme abnormalities arose as a result of regressive changes that took place subsequent to a process of maturation, which was in itself not abnormal.

IV. Cardio-Myopathy of the Syrian Hamster

In studies on skeletal muscle in the <u>hereditary cardio-myopathy of the Syrian hamster</u> (<u>Mesocricetus auratus</u>)(16, 17, 152, 163) hyperbasophilia of the sarcoplasm as related to mitochondrial content of muscle fibres was observed in carrier animals. This finding could indicate a predominant involvement of (red) type-1 fibres in this disease. Accordingly, and in contrast to the findings in dystrophic mice (114), the ventricular myocardium of the diseased animals was severely affected (216), showing signs of delayed maturation (47) such as large numbers of ribosomes, poorly oriented myofilaments, mitotic figures (224) and a small-sized fetal type of mitochondria (279).

Summarizing, it can be stated that in the hereditary myopathies of mouse, chicken and hamster, in the (neuro-)myopathy of vincristine and, with certain limitations, in the myopathy of vitamin-E deficiency in rat and rabbit, white (type-2) fibres in skeletal muscle are predilectively affected. Findings in corticosteroid myopathy are to some degree ambiguous, yet there is evidence that type-2 (white) fibres are also predominantly involved. Accordingly, in myopathies of this type the myocardium, which is a red muscle, is completely spared or only slightly affected. On the other hand, in the myopathy of chloroquine and presumably in the cardio-myopathy of the Syrian hamster, red (type-1) muscle fibres are predominantly involved and the heart muscle is severely affected.

There is thus considerable evidence to suggest that the dystrophic process becomes manifest in skeletal muscle at a period when white (type-2) muscle fibres differentiate from the ontogenetically preceding fetal red muscle fibres.

The Myopathy of 2,4-Dichlorophenoxyacetic Acid (2,4-D) in the Rat

The myopathy elicited by the herbicide 2,4-dichlorophenoxyacetic acid (2,4-D) is another example of predilective involvement of white (type-2) muscle fibres in an experimental disease. By appropriate dosage of this agent, acute or subacute myopathic states can be evoked in warm-blooded animals. The principal subject of the present study is the subacute myopathy of 2,4-D induced in the white rat by repeated injections of the substance. Preceding this section, the results of a critical re-evaluation (139, 141) of the sequelae of acute intoxication with 2,4-D are discussed.

Material, Methods and Remarks

A. Treatment of Animals

I. In-Vitro Experiments (vt)

These experiments were performed on sections from the triceps surae and tibialis anterior muscles of normal Wistar rats, 160 to 170 g in weight. For
details of animal conditions, preparation of muscle samples and technique
of sectioning see paragraph III.

II. In-Vivo Experiments with Acute Intoxication (avi)

One to 1.5 h before being decapitated, Wistar rats weighing 160 to 170 g were
given under slight ether narcosis a single intraperitoneal injection of
300 mg/kg of 2,4-D. This dosage corresponds to one quarter to one half of
the LD_{50} (69, refs.). Controls were given an equal amount of physiological
saline. In the experimental animals marked adynamia and myotonia developed
within 30 min and were still present at the time of decapitation. In sur-
viving animals this acute syndrome was observed to decline almost completely within 5 to 6 h. One day after a single injection of 300 mg/kg of 2,4-D
the animals had fully recovered.

III. In-Vivo Experiments with Subacute Intoxication (svi)

The experiments were carried out from mid-May to mid-November on female
Wistar rats, 160 to 170 g of weight (S. Ivanovas, Kisslegg, Allgäu, FRG).
The animals were kept in an air-conditioned room in normal daylight. They
received Altromin and water ad lib. Daily at 7 to 8 a.m. the experimental
animals were given, under slight ether narcosis, intraperitoneal injections
of 100 to 150 mg/kg of 2,4-D which had been isotonically dissolved in sodium
bicarbonate (139). For details of treatment, see Table 1. Corresponding to
the severity of the developing clinical condition, the doses of 2,4-D were
varied from 80 to 100 mg/kg per day. Changes in body weight, delay in muscular relaxation following the jerk of the anterior tibial muscle, and the
time course of posture reflexes from a given dorsal position were qualitative criteria of the action of 2,4-D. Treatment was continued at maximum
up to the critical reduction of 30% of initial weight. This point was
generally reached on the first day after a continued treatment of 13 days.
At this time, a marked myotonic-myopathic syndrome was present. The animals
reacted only weakly to stimuli and transiently took no food. On trying to
walk, they dragged their hind legs, which were always more markedly affected than the forelegs. When the anterior tibial jerk was elicited, subsequent

Table 1. Subacute intoxication with 2,4-D (svi). Dosage and course of treatment as reflected in decrease of body weight (C = Controls; E = Experimental animals)

Animal	Initial weight (g)	Terminal weight (g)	% change of body weight	Days of treatment (n)	% of maximal weight loss during treatment	Days of survival after treatment	Total dose of 2,4-D (g/kg)	Mean single dose of 2,4-D (g/kg/day)	Animal killed during P=progression[a] R=remission[a]
C_1	215	?	?	3 (NaCl)	–	0	–	–	indifferent
C_2	235	250	+ 6.4	10 (NaCl)	–	13	–	–	indifferent
C_3	140	160	+ 14.2	11 (NaCl)	–	0	–	–	indifferent
C_4	140	205	+ 46.3	17 (NaCl)	–	2	–	–	indifferent
C_5	145	225	+ 55.0	33 (NaCl)	–	1	–	–	indifferent
C_6	175	180	+ 2.9	4 (NaCl)	–	1	–	–	indifferent
C_7	170	210	+ 23.5	12 (NaCl)	–	11	–	–	indifferent
C_8	155	195	+ 25.8	12 (NaCl)	–	15	–	–	indifferent
E_1	240	255	+ 6.30	6	6.25	0	0.500	0.083	P
E_2	160	150	– 6.30	11	9.35	0	1.50	0.14	P
E_3	150	135	– 10.00	10	33.3	1	1.25	0.13	P
E_4	155	125	– 19.3	17	32.4	2	2.20	0.13	P
E_5	155	185	+ 19.3	33	6.45	1	4.44	0.134	P
E_6	170	140	– 17.6	4	17.6	1	0.50	0.125	P
E_7	230	230	± 0	14	21.8	13	1.10	0.09	R
E_8	220	210	– 4.55	14	20.5	13	1.10	0.09	R
E_9	160	140	– 12.5	7	12.5	1	0.750	0.11	R
E_{10}	165	155	– 6.1	7	39.4	16	0.750	0.11	R
E_{11}	175	190	+ 8.55	12	28.6	15	1.60	0.13	R

[a] of myopathy.

relaxation was markedly delayed, as were the posture reflexes. On being
lifted from the floor by the tail, the animals failed to stretch and, when
lowered to the floor again, did not show a supporting reaction. At this stage
of the disease, treatment was halted and spontaneous recovery was expected.
During treatment, some animals showed transient signs of capillary haemorrhage
with clotting of blood at their lid margins. This symptom was constantly
present in the avi experiments. Control animals were treated in a similar
manner with physiological saline. They showed no impairment, their body
weight increasing continuously to 12 to 15% of the initial weight during
the experimental period. Results were obtained from 8 control and 11 experimental animals at various stages of the disease (see Table 1).

B.   Preparation of Samples

After decapitation, the spinal cord was immediately destroyed by use of a
probe introduced into the spinal channel. This was done in order to abolish
spinal reflexes which might give rise to postmortal metabolic changes in the
corresponding muscles. A sample of liver, the heart and the triceps surae
muscle were quickly removed and, until further preparation could be performed, were stored at 4°C for up to 5 min in Ringer's solution. Appropriate
pieces of each organ were, in the sequence of their excision, trimmed in
cooled Ringer's solution, put on a chuck of the cryostat microtome and
chilled in propane cooled by liquid nitrogen (-165°C). Cracks in the tissue
sample due to chilling were soldered with ice water at the base of samples
(139). Sections, 10 μm in thickness were cut on the microtome at -25° to
-20°C. Three sections from each liver and muscle and two from the heart
were melted on cooled cover slides and stored in the cryostat prior to
histochemical processing. Maximum time of storage was up to 30 h at -30°C
and adequate humidity. By systematically processing two to three sections
per cover slide, unspecific differences in histochemical reactivity could
be eliminated. The histochemical reactions were performed in each case on
a cover slide taken from the beginning and on one taken from the end of
the series; thus 4 to 6 sections were processed per reaction. No loss of
enzyme activities was observed within the series.

C.   Staining Procedures and Histochemical Reactions

The modified trichrome stain was used for skeletal muscle (100), and the
hematoxylin-eosin stain for heart and liver. Glycogen was demonstrated by
use of the alcoholic variant of the PAS reaction (MCMANUS, 1946 (233)),
RNS was demonstrated with methyl green-pyronine (BRACHET, 1942 (233)) and
the Sudan III-IV stain was used to visualize lipids (KAY and WHITEHEAD,
1941 (233)). The calcium-cobalt method (226) with differentiating preincubations of the sections in buffer solutions (pH 9.4, 4.5, 4.3 (37, 38))
was applied in the demonstration of myofibrillar ATPase. Preincubations
were performed for 5 min and incubations for 25 to 30 min at 20 to 22°C.
All the histological and histochemical reactions were done in mounted
cryostat sections.

I. Histochemical Demonstration of Phosphorylase and Glycogen Synthetase. Suggestions and Remarks

In earlier experiments on sections of skeletal muscle of normal animals, a decrease in phosphorylase activity had been observed when 2,4-D was incorporated into the aqueous incubation solution (139). Since the possibility of a diffusion of newly synthesized amylopectin and of phosphorylase from the section into the incubation medium could not be ruled out, the results did not strictly prove inhibition of the enzyme by 2,4-D. ECKNER et al. (84) critically reviewed the problems involved in the histochemical demonstration of phosphorylase by means of both aqueous and modified viscous incubation solutions (207, 208). In order to diminish the loss of enzyme from the section during incubation, PETTE and co-workers designed for quantitative histo- and biochemical studies incubation media containing polyacrylamide (239, 271). By supplying auxiliary enzymes and NBT they succeeded in demonstrating phosphorylase indirectly by means of a stable end-product, which is diformazane. The original methods (155, 291, 292, 293) provided direct demonstration of amylopectin by means of the iodine stain. The indirect methods for the demonstration of phosphorylase were not applied in the present study, first, because they are rather tedious in routine histochemistry and, second, because the earlier results (139) had been obtained by means of the standard reactions (291, 292). It was attempted in the present study to combine the advantage of a direct demonstration of amylopectin with that of a diminished enzyme efflux from the sections during incubation. This was effected by changing the substrate concentrations and by incorporating 3% of gelatin into the aqueous incubation media. For a critical evaluation of the results, serial sections were incubated in parallel for phosphorylase and for glycogen synthetase, in both gelatin and aqueous media of the following compositions (end concentrations in brackets):

Phosphorylase:

Gelat. Incub. Med.		Aqueous Incub. Med.
80 mg (21.2 mM)	G1P[1]	40 mg (10.6 mM)
80 mg (21.5 mM)	EDTA	75 mg (20.2 mM)
20 mg (48 mM)	NaF	10 mg (24 mM)
10 mg (5 mM)	MgCl$_2$	5 mg (2.5 mM)
10 mg (2.9 mM)	cAMP 0.1M	5 mg (1.44 mM)
5 ml	Acet. buffer pH 5.9	10 ml
5 ml	Acetate Gelat. 6%, pH 5.9	

---

[1] Abbreviations: ATPase = adenosine-5'-triphosphatase; LDH = lactate dehydrogenase; m-GDH = menadione-dependent glycerine-1-phosphate dehydrogenase; NAD = nicotineamide-adenine-dinucleotide; NADP = nicotineamide-adenine-dinucleotide-phosphate; SDH = succinodehydrogenase; G-6-PDH = glucose-6-phosphate dehydrogenase; phosphorylase = α-1,4-glucane:orthophosphate glucosyltransferase; UDPG-GT = uridine-diphosphate-glucose glucosyltransferase, glycogen synthetase; NBT = nitro-blue tetrazoliumchloride; NADH-TR = NADH-tetrazolium reductase; G-1-P = glucose-1-phosphate; cAMP = adenosine-3',5'-monophosphate, cyclic; EDTA = ethylenediaminetetraacetic acid; UDPG = uridine-5'-diphosphoglucose.

Glycogen Synthetase:
____

50 mg (8.2 mM)	UDPG	25 mg (4.1 mM)
20 mg (6.6 mM)	G6P	10 mg (3.3 mM)
60 mg (16 mM)	EDTA	56 mg (15 mM)
5 ml	0.2 M Tris Buffer pH 7.4	10 ml
5 ml	Tris Gelat. 6%, pH 7.4	

Aqueous incubations were performed without preceding freeze-substitution in
a modified Hori medium (155). The pH of all the aqueous solutions was ad-
justed immediately prior to incubation or to the addition of gelatin, respectively. 6% gelatin (powdered) was dissolved in 0.1 M acetate buffer (pH =
5.9 for phosphorylase) or in 0.2 M Tris buffer (pH = 7.4 for glycogen synthetase). The gelatin incubation films were prepared by dropping a sufficient
amount of liquid gelatin medium upon cool cover slides to form a film some
2 mm thick. The slides were stored for about 10 min in a refrigerator until
the films had become sufficiently solid. The mounted cryostat sections were
then put into contact with the surface of the films. Incubation was performed at 22°C, and was 3 and 5 h for phosphorylase and glycogen synthetase,
respectively. At this time, the sets were cooled as mentioned and the mounted
sections were carefully removed from their films. With these precautions,
gelatin was never observed to adhere to the sections. These were immediately
fixed in 100% propanol for 5 min and stored along with their gelatin films
at 4°C until the microscopic examination could be done.

Unfixed cryostat sections were incubated in parallel in the aqueous solution
at 34°C over periods of 40 and 120 min for phosphorylase and glycogen synthetase, respectively. The sections were then briefly rinsed in 40% propanol,
air-dried and fixed in 100% alcohol.

Newly formed amylopectin was invariably demonstrated by means of Gram's iodine.
The PAS reaction served as control. The iodine-staining process has the advantage that it provides a fair distinction between the different forms of
long-chain "blue", and of branched or low-molecular "brownish" amylopectin
(289). Primary glycogen does not stain specifically with iodine and was demonstrated by means of the PAS-reaction. Unincubated fixed sections and sections incubated in the absence of substrate served as controls. The newly
formed amylopectin could be sufficiently characterized by comparing the results of the iodine and of the PAS-staining. Thus an identification by means
of the diastase reaction proved unnecessary.

The in vitro effects of 2,4-D were studied by dissolving 14 mM of the substance (sodium salt, (139)) in the aqueous or gelatin incubation medium at
constant pH. As stated above, the gelatin techniques for the demonstration
of the enzymes of glycogen metabolism were used particularly for the in-vitro
and the acute in-vivo (vt and avi) experiments. Since in the latter, as well
as in the experiments with subacute intoxication (svi), no qualitative differences in reactivity between the aqueous and the gelatin incubations could
be observed in the sections, only the aqueous technique was used to study
the changes of subacute intoxication.

II. NAD- and NADP-Dependent Dehydrogenases. Remarks and Methods

Activities of these enzymes were determined by means of gelatin incubation media without addition of phenazinemethosulfate (PMS). Gelatin incubation media impede the efflux of enzymes from the section and thus improve localization (105, 106). Addition of the electron carrier PMS to the histochemical dehydrogenase incubation solutions will shunt the action of diaphorases present in the tissue (31, 300). In standard histochemical media without PMS, these enzymes will limit the activities of the specific dehydrogenases. PMS, by effecting the direct transfer of hydrogen ions from the reduced coenzyme (NADH or NADPH) to the acceptor molecule (NBT), renders the histochemical reaction independent of tissue diaphorase.

The finding that the histochemical activity of lactate dehydrogenase (without PMS in the incubation solution) is higher in red than in white muscle fibres can be explained by the fact that the limiting activities of NADH-diaphorase are low in white and high in red muscle cells. As established in biochemical studies, the lactate dehydrogenase activity of white muscle fibres is actually higher than that of red fibres (27, 31). Hence the histochemical pattern of lactate dehydrogenase represents the true activity of the diaphorase and not that of LDH. The addition of PMS to the histochemical incubation media was an attempt to bridge the gap between the histochemical and biochemical findings, at least on the semiquantitative scale (239, 300). However, depending upon the PMS concentrations used in the experiments, it is possible to produce a histochemical pattern varying from the standard picture up to the point of complete inversion (35, 36, 112, 137, 197). At given concentrations of PMS, any desired pattern of fibre type staining can be produced by changing the substrate concentrations in the incubation solutions (35, 36). These findings suggest that the quantitative reduction of NBT to formazan by means of PMS is impeded by a shunt in the reaction chain, due possibly to the different activities of cytochrome oxidase in red and white muscle fibres. These results show that the differences induced by PMS in the histochemical lactate dehydrogenase activities can only be regarded with reservations as representing the actual activity of LDH in the muscle fibres. In addition, according to our own experience, considerable formazan production occurred in histochemical media containing PMS in the absence of enzyme, even when kept in darkness. Finally, the histochemical staining of cytological details was not satisfactory.

Because of these objections, gelatinous incubation media were applied without PMS to the histochemical demonstration of dehydrogenase activities. The limitations mentioned above, due to the diaphorase present in the tissue, were taken into account, but diffusion of enzyme and of formazan from the section was markedly diminished as against aqueous media. When this method is used, quantitative statements concerning the respective enzyme activities are necessarily confined to the biochemical field of investigation.

The gelatinous incubation media had the following composition:

Substrate (1 M, pH 7.2)[a]	0.6 ml	(0.215 mM)
MgCl$_2$ (0.05 M, pH 7.2)[b]	0.4 ml	(7.15 mM)
NaN$_3$ (0.15 M, pH 7.2)	0.2 ml	(7.0 mM)
NBT (2 mg/ml, pH 7.2)	0.3 ml	(0.27 mM)
NAD	3.5 mg	(1.9 mM)
or NADP	3.5 mg	(1.6 mM)
or menadione[c]	3.5 mg	(7.25 mM)
Tris-HCl-Buffer (0.2 M, pH 7.2)	1.3 ml	(0.26 mM)

[a] Succinate stock solution:pH 7.4.

[b] Ommitted in the medium for SDH.

[c] For the demonstration of m-GDH.

Succinate, α-glycerophosphate, glucose-6-phosphate and lactate served as substrates.

The aqueous phase of the incubation solution was mixed with an equal amount of slightly warmed 6% gelatin in 0.2 M Tris buffer (pH 7.2 or 7.4, respectively). The coenzyme (NAD, NADP, menadione) was added immediately prior to incubation. Clouding of the incubation solution for m-GDH when menadione was added did not interfere with the histochemical reaction. Complete incubation media were dropped directly onto cold, unfixed cryostat sections. Incubation was performed for 60 to 90 min at 20°C in a moist chamber. The result of the histochemical reaction was observed under the microscope during incubation. There was neither evidence of the formation of formazan in the incubation medium apart from the section, nor of diffusion of the reaction product from the sections into the gelatinous medium. At the end of the incubation period the gelatinous film was carefully washed off in hand-warm water. Sections were then taken through graded acetone water mixtures (99). By this procedure, both monoformazan, corresponding to the sites of minor enzyme activity, and formazan, which is bound to lipids, will be dissolved, whereas the sites of high enzyme activity, corresponding to the formation of insoluble blue diformazan, become more distinct. Sections were enclosed in Kayser's glycerogel.

Under the conditions defined above, the histochemical dehydrogenase reactions were used in the first instance as a staining for the demonstration of cytological details and of the earliest alterations in the muscle cell. As such, histochemical reactions can complete and extend the reliability of the histological stainings. Statements as to differences in the histochemical reactivity of the sections were always referred to the comparison of sections from experimental and from control animals.

Fibre Types of Normal Skeletal Muscle

From the physiological, biochemical and histochemical points of
view, the historical distinction of "red" and "white" muscle
fibres as derived from the macroscopical appearance of muscles
(95, refs.) must nowadays be regarded as inadequate. Evidence
obtained from experiments with cross-innervation of muscle indicated that the differentiation of fibre types in skeletal
muscle is controlled by trophic influences of nerve on muscle
(25, 48, 126, 128). It has been further demonstrated (86, 151)
that in the course of physiological training of muscle over
long periods of time, as well as in experimental animals receiv-
ing hormonal treatment, the criteria of fibre types in skeletal
muscle can be shifted towards an increase in oxidative (mitochondrial) enzyme activities (143, refs.). The characteristics
of muscle fibre types can thus be modified by different physiological conditions.

The various fibre types of skeletal muscle can be distinguished
essentially by means of two histochemical reactions, the reaction for myosin-ATPase with preincubations (38), and the mitochondrial dehydrogenase reactions, in particular that of NADH-
tetrazolium reductase (NADH-TR). The phosphorylase reaction is
also useful for this purpose (78). Different cytological structures are involved in these procedures. The standard ATPase
reaction enables two fibre types to be distinguished (226):
type-1 fibres with weak reactivity, and type-2 fibres with strong
reactivity. This classification does not clearly coincide with
the notion that red and white are correlated with the mitochondrial content of the respective muscle fibres.

A relationship was found to exist between the ATPase type of
muscle fibre on the one hand and contraction velocity and fatigability upon repeated stimulation on the other. Fast contracting
fibres with a high rate of fatigability are type-2, whereas slowly contracting fibres which sustain contractility over long periods are type-1 fibres (26, 51). In agreement with this, the
biochemical activity of myosin ATPase was found to increase in
parallel with the maximal contraction speed of a given muscle
fibre (24, 25, 212). Characteristic differences in the acid-
base stability of myosin ATPase serve to distinguish subtypes
A, B and C of the main type-2 fibre (38, 127, 259, 316); these
are not identical with the mitochondrial types of A, B and C
fibres (see below).

Preference is given in fibre typing to the myosin ATPase reaction because it proves remarkably constant in different physio-

logical and pathological conditions of the muscle fibre, in particular in neurogenic atrophy. Thus, following experimental denervation of muscle, this reaction provided adequate typing of muscle fibres for up to 27 weeks after nerve section (174) whereas by this time, the original fibre type could no longer be assessed by means of the mitochondrial reactions.

By increasing the number of histochemical reactions applied to serial sections, up to 8 fibre types could be discerned in cat muscle (247). It must, however, be admitted that actual differences in the physiological activity of motor units might be reflected in this number (86, 151, 179, 181). This applies in particular to differences in glycogen content and phosphorylase activity in the muscle fibres. Three fibre types can be distinguished by means of the NADH-TR reaction (Figs. 1 and 2): white A_m fibres with low mitochondrial content, intermediate or B_m fibres, and red or C_m fibres, rich in mitochondria (281).[2]

As viewed with the electron microscope, the fibres of these three types present typical cytological differences (225).

EDGERTON and co-workers have elucidated, in experimental work on the guinea pig, the relations between histochemical, biochemical and contractile properties of the three fibre types (26, 85, 87, 88).

These are as follows:

1. fast-twitch white (A_m) fibres with a low mitochondrial content and with high myosin ATPase activity. They correspond to the ATPase subtype 2B (38).

2. fast-twitch red (C_m) fibres with high mitochondrial content and high ATPase activity, corresponding to the ATPase subtype 2A (38) and

3. slow-twitch intermediate (B_m) fibres with high mitochondrial content and low ATPase activity, corresponding to ATPase type-1.

Hence, having regard to the type of the $2A/C_m$ fibre, it cannot be claimed that red muscle fibres would as a rule be slowly contracting fibres (26).

In order to obtain a sufficient discrimination of fibre types in skeletal muscle, at least two histochemical reactions ought to be performed: the (differential) reaction(s) for ATPase (38) and that for NADH-TR. In the present study, the discrimination of fibre types was based on these two reactions, and in particular on the ATPase reaction with differentiating preincubations (38). This proved important, in particular as regards the com-

---

[2] In the present study, the index$_m$ (= mitochondrial) is used throughout, to characterize the mitochondrial fibre type. Fibres are listed according to their ATPase/NADH-TR reactions, e.g. $2B/A_m$.

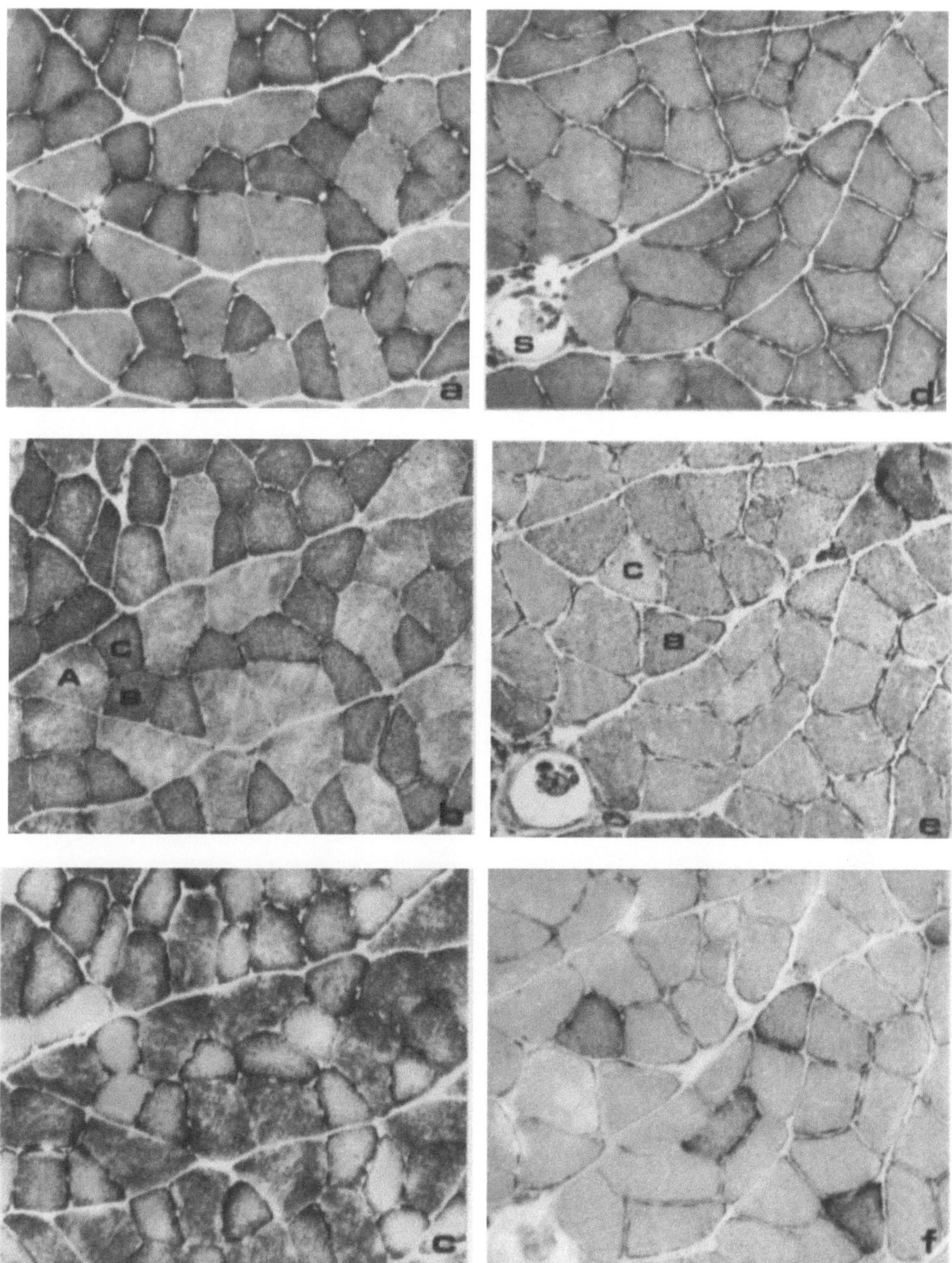

Fig. 1a-f. Histochemical reactions and fibre types in the skeletal muscle of the normal rat. (a-c): M. gastrocnemius, mid layer; (d-f): M. soleus. Serial sections. (a) and (d): modified trichrome; (b) and (e): NADH-TR; (c) and (f): menadione-mediated GDH. (b) and (e): mitochondrial fibre types A, B, and C (= A_m, B_m, C_m, see text). Increased subsarcolemmal reaction of C_m compared with B_m fibres with the menadione-GDH reaction (c) and (f). Minor differences in the reactivity of B_m and C_m fibres of the soleus muscle (e). S = muscle spindle. x 180. See also Fig. 2

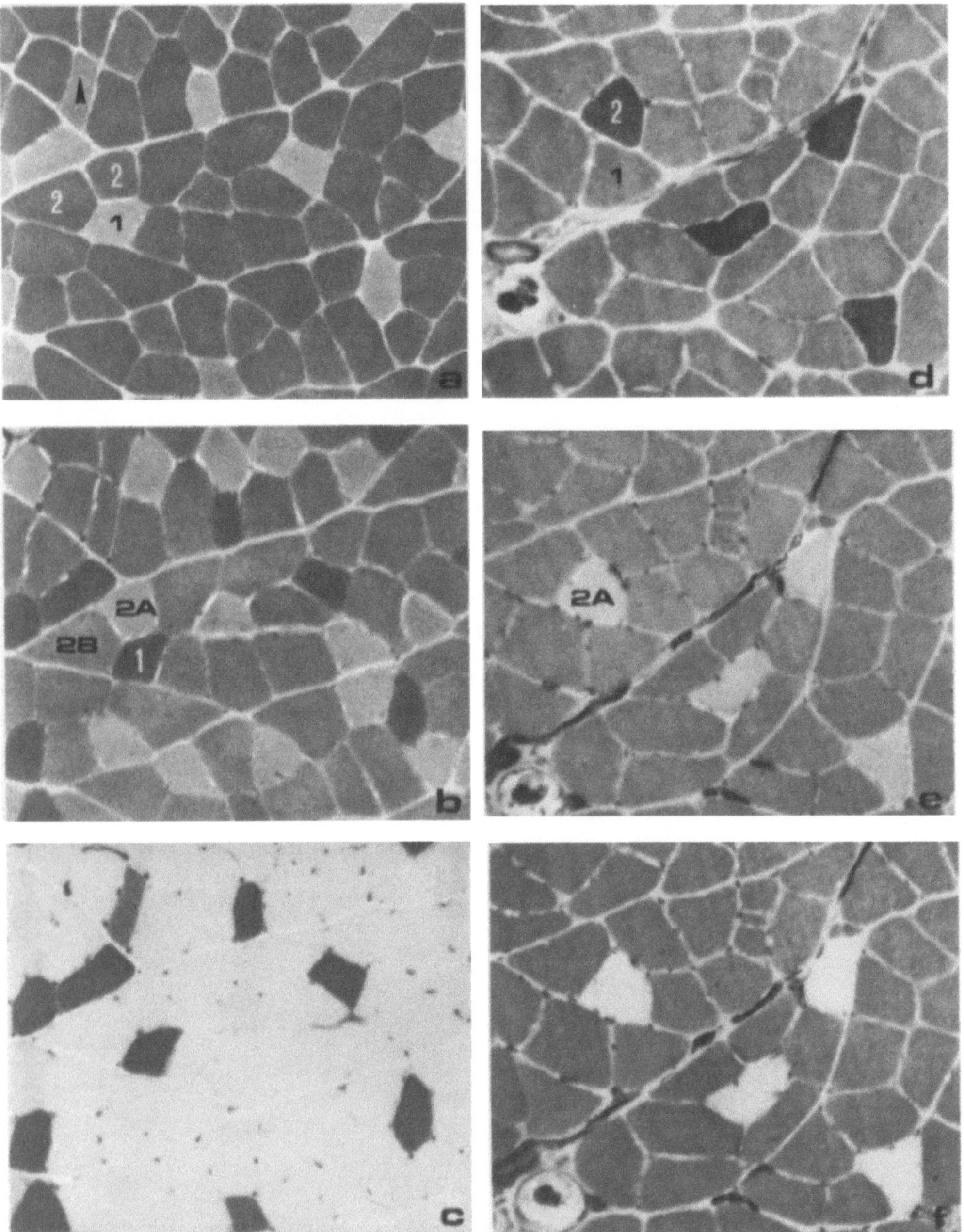

Fig. 2a-f. Myosin-ATPase reaction with preincubations. (a) and
(d): pH 9.4; (b) and (e): pH 4.6; (c) and (f): pH 4.3. Inversion
of the reaction pattern from (a-c) and from (d-f). Two fibre types
can be discerned with preincubation at pH 9.4, three fibre types
at pH 4.6: types 1, 2A and 2B. ▲ = type-2C fibre with a positive
reaction over the whole pH range. Serial sections to Fig. 1.
x 180

parison of our data with those in other experimental conditions
and with the results obtained in studies of muscle biopsies in
man. In addition the menadione-mediated GDH reaction played an
equally important role in the demonstration of cytological details, as did the PAS-reaction for glycogen and the demonstration of phosphorylase, especially under pathological conditions.
A survey of the reactions is given in Table 2 and in Figs. 1
and 2.

A quantitative estimate of the regional distribution of the
three fibre types shows that in the superficial parts of the
gastrocnemius muscle (medial head) the vast majority of fibres
are $2B/A_m$ fibres, whereas in the deeper layers the predominant
$2B/A_m$ fibres are intermingled with $2A/C_m$ and $1/B_m$ fibres. The
deepest regions of this muscle, adjacent to the soleus muscle,
are composed of fairly equal parts of type-2 (A_m and C_m) and
of type-1/B_m fibres; ATPase type-2A fibres outnumber 2B-fibres
here. The bulk of the fibres of the soleus are type-1/B_m,
followed by a small amount of $2A/C_m$ and a negligible proportion of $2B/A_m$ fibres. Lowest activities of NADH-TR can be observed in the true white $2B/A_m$ fibre of the gastrocnemius
muscle. The tibialis anterior, like the superficial parts of
the gastrocnemius, is composed for up to two thirds of its
thickness of $2B/A_m$ and sparse $2A/C_m$ fibres. The fibre type
pattern of the deep region of the anterior tibial muscle
corresponds to that of the mid-layer of the gastrocnemius.

Table 2. Histochemical characteristics of muscle fibres of the gastrocnemius and soleus muscles of the rat

| Reaction | soleus | | gastrocnemius | | | fibre type: |
	red high, type C_m type 2A	intermediate interm., type B_m type 1	red high, type C_m type 2A	intermediate interm., type B_m type 1	white low, type A_m type 2B	general denomination mitochondrial content myosin-ATPase
ATPase pH 9.4/4.5/4.3	++/∅/∅	∅/+(+)/++	++/∅/∅	∅/+(+)/++	++/(+)/∅	
NADH–TR (LDH)	++	+(+)[a]	++	+(+)	(+)	
SDH	+(+)	+[a]	+(+)	+	(+)	
men–GDH	(+)	∅	+[a]	(+) or ∅	++	
Phosphorylase[b]	+ brown-violet	+(+) brown	+ brown	+ brown-violet	+ blue-violet	
Glycogen synthetase	+ brown	(+) brown	+ brown	(+) brown	∅	
Glycogen	(+)	(+)	+	(+)	++	

[a] activity accentuated in the subsarcolemmal space.

[b] incubation without addition of ethanol. Subsequent iodine stain.

(+) low; + intermediate; ++ high activity.

Results

A. Effects of 2,4-D in vitro on the Histochemical Reaction for Phosphorylase in Skeletal Muscle (vt). Results and Discussion

As can be seen from Table 3, the results of the earlier experiments were confirmed. These indicate (139) that the phosphorylase reaction in the sections will be inhibited if the aqueous incubation is performed in the presence of 2,4-D at a concentration of 14 mM (S_a in Table 3). The same applies to the phosphorylase reaction in the gelatin films into which 2,4-D has been incorporated (G_g). In striking contrast to this, no apparent decrease of phosphorylase activity can be observed in the corresponding sections (S_g). As shown in the earlier experiments with aqueous incubation (139), the activity of glycogen synthetase does not, in fact, change in the presence of 2,4-D in the gelatin film.

Table 3. Effects of 2,4-D (14 mM) on the histochemical reaction for phosphorylase in sections of skeletal muscle (triceps surae, tibialis anterior)

	O mM 2,4-D	14 mM 2,4-D
G_g	++	Ø
S_g	++	++
S_a	++	Ø

G_g = gelatin films (separated from corresponding sections S_g).
S_g = sections from gelatinous incubations.
S_a = sections from aqueous incubations.

It can be concluded from the results in Table 3 that during incubation some of the enzyme and/or newly formed amylopectin can diffuse out of the sections into the gelatin film (see G_g at O mM of 2,4-D). The contrast between the positive phosphorylase reaction in the sections (S_g) of the gelatinous incubation in the presence of 2,4-D (14 mM) and the negative reaction in the corresponding films (G_g = 14 mM) suggests that after a certain period of incubation the section is no longer accessible to sufficient 2,4-D to exert detectable inhibition on the synthesis of amylopectin. Inhibition of this process does occur, however, in the gelatin film with incorporated 2,4-D (14 mM); in this case, phosphorylase activity diffusing off the sections is inhibited. Hypothetical masking of amylopectin by 2,4-D, resulting in a negative iodine reaction in the gelatin film, could hardly account for these findings, which are highly suggestive of a block in the synthesis of amylopectin due to inhibition at some stage in the phosphorylase activating system.

The results of aqueous incubations are in agreement with these interpretations. In spite of uncontrolled loss of phosphorylase and amylopectin into the aqueous incubation solution, the amount of enzyme retained in the section can be markedly inhibited by 2,4-D, which, in the aqueous solution, is freely diffusible. Since, in the gelatin film with incorporated 2,4-D, the phosphorylase reaction is negative, it cannot be concluded that 2,4-D would act by increasing the efflux of enzyme and/or of amylopectin from the section. The opposite assumption, that the only effect of 2,4-D is to impede the efflux of enzyme and of amylopectin from the section, is clearly contradicted by the decreased activity of phosphorylase in sections incubated with 2,4-D in the aqueous solution (S_a 14 mM).

The results of the gelatin film incubations on the whole confirm earlier findings obtained with aqueous incubation media (139), indicating that, histochemically, the activity of muscle phosphorylase is diminished by 2,4-D. Biochemically, no specific inhibition of phosphorylase a or b by 2,4-D was demonstrated (110), therefore it is likely that the decrease in phosphorylase activity is brought about by 2,4-D effecting inhibition at some stage of the phosphorylase activating system (180, refs., 144).

Comparable findings, i.e. a significant decrease of phosphorylase activity in the stalk and leaves of red beans consequent to local treatment with 2,4-D, have been demonstrated biochemically by NEELY et al. (217).

B. Effects of Acute Intoxication in vivo on the Glycogen Metabolism of Skeletal Muscle (avi). Histochemical Findings and Discussion

The results obtained on skeletal muscle with aqueous and gelatin film incubations following acute intoxication of the animals with 2,4-D (300 mg/kg i.p.) were qualitatively similar for both the triceps surae and the anterior tibial muscles. Hence, only the results of the gelatin film incubations will be considered here, since they are more conclusive on a semi-quantitative scale. The changes differed markedly in the two muscles in quality and amount. Phosphorylase activity was found to be only slightly and inconstantly diminished in sections from the triceps surae muscle of treated animals. The intensity of the iodine stain in the corresponding films did not differ from that of controls. It can be stated that, at the time at which this muscle was excised, it was impossible to ascertain any overall decrease in phosphorylase activity in the sections, nor could differences be established in the efflux of enzyme and amylopectin (Fig. 3). The only changes comparable to those observed in the anterior tibial

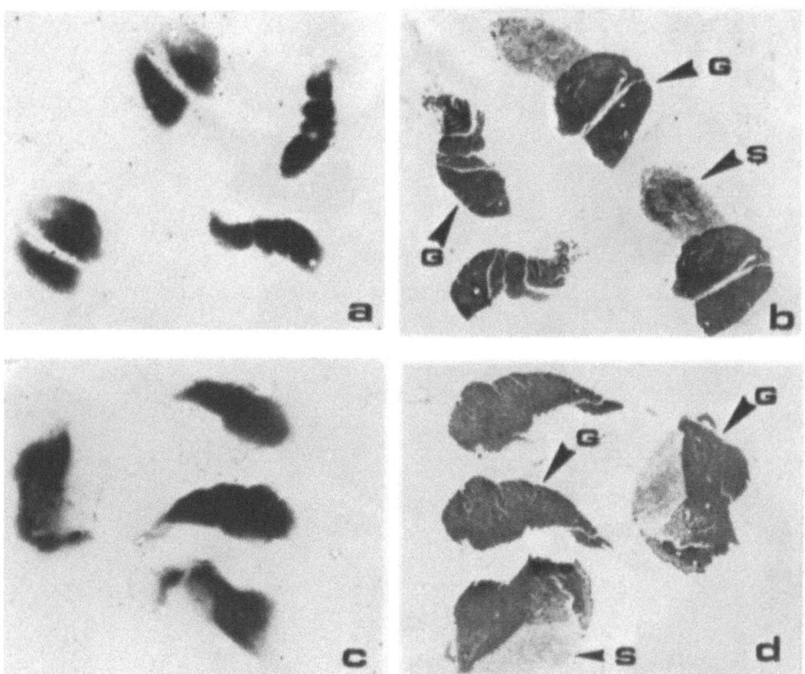

Fig. 3a-d. Triceps surae, acute intoxication (avi). Phosphorylase reaction, gelatinous incubation technique. (a) and (c):
reaction in the gelatin films; (b) and (d): reactions in the
corresponding sections. (a) and (b): controls; (c) and (d):
1 h following i.p. injection of 300 mg/kg 2,4-D. G = gastrocnemius, S = soleus. Slight decrease in the activity of the
gastrocnemius in treated animals (b) and (d) without significant
differences in the corresponding gelatin films (a) and (c).
No demonstrable efflux of activity from the soleus into the
gelatin film. x 3.3

muscle occurred in the deeper layers of the calf muscle. These
are composed of typical $2A/C_m$ fibres and of morphologically
slightly different $2A/C_m$ fibres of the soleus type (Figs. 1,
2, and 5). In treated animals, some of these fibres displayed
increased phosphorylase activity as shown by an intensified
brownish reaction with iodine (Fig. 5). Increased amounts of
primary glycogen could be demonstrated in these cells as
opposed to neighbouring $2B/A_m$ fibres; a considerable proportion of the latter stained positive for phosphorylase, but
negative for primary glycogen. A marked overall decrease in
phosphorylase activity together with loss of primary glycogen
from the muscle cell was observed in the anterior tibial muscle
(Fig. 4). Additional differences in enzyme activity could be
demonstrated between the superficial and mid-layers (consisting
of $2B/A_m$ and of sparse $2A/C_m$ fibres) of this muscle and its
deepest parts (composed of 2B, 2A and type-1 fibres)(Fig. 6).
Thus the relatively homogeneous and moderate iodine stain for
phosphorylase in the outer and mid-zone of the sections con-
trasted with an almost negative reaction in the corresponding

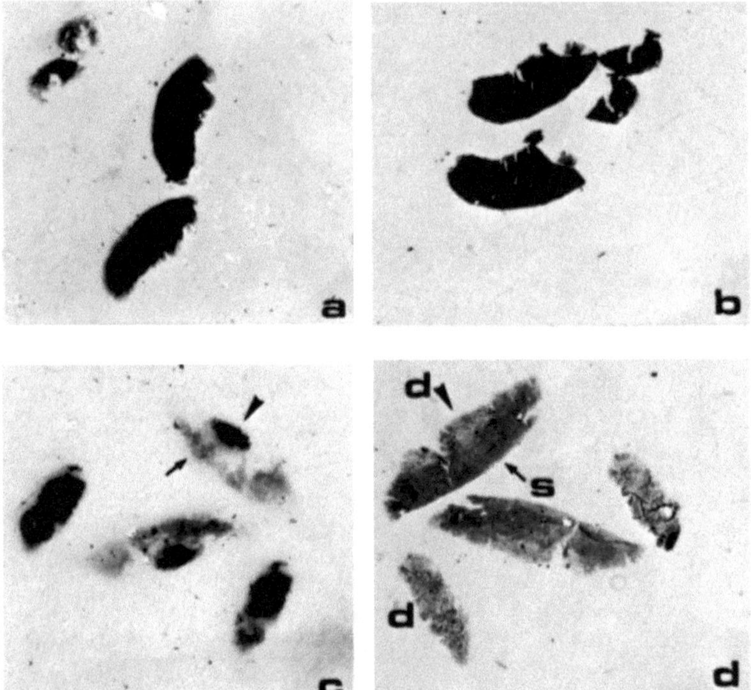

Fig. 4a-d. Tibialis anterior, acute intoxication (avi). Animals and sequence of pictures same as in Fig. 3. s = superficial, d = deep layer of the muscle. Corresponding sites in sections and in gelatin films are marked by arrows. Marked overall decrease in phosphorylase activity, in particular in the deep layer of the muscle of treated animals (d) as compared to the gastrocnemius (Fig. 3). Sites of maximum activity in the gelatin film correspond to sites of minimal enzyme activity in the section and vice versa (see arrows). x 3.3

areas of the gelatin film, and inhomogeneously distributed weak or zero activities of the enzyme in the deep layers of muscle were opposed to strong positive reactions in the corresponding film, yielding a blue-violet stain (Fig. 4). These findings are listed in Table 4 and illustrated by Fig. 5.

The principal findings, loss of phosphorylase activity and of primary glycogen, were observed in almost half the $2B/A_m$ fibres, one fifth of the $2A/C_m$ fibres and two fifths of the sparse $1/B_m$ fibres. In addition, as with the findings in the deep layer of the gastrocnemius, an increase in phosphorylase activity occurred in more than one fourth of $2A/C_m$ and one twentieth of $2B/A_m$ fibres. Fibres of these types characteristically displayed increased amounts of primary glycogen and atypically increased activities of NADH-TR. A proportion of $2B/A_m$ fibres was not involved in these changes; some of these displayed negative reactions for glycogen and a positive reaction for phosphorylase (87).

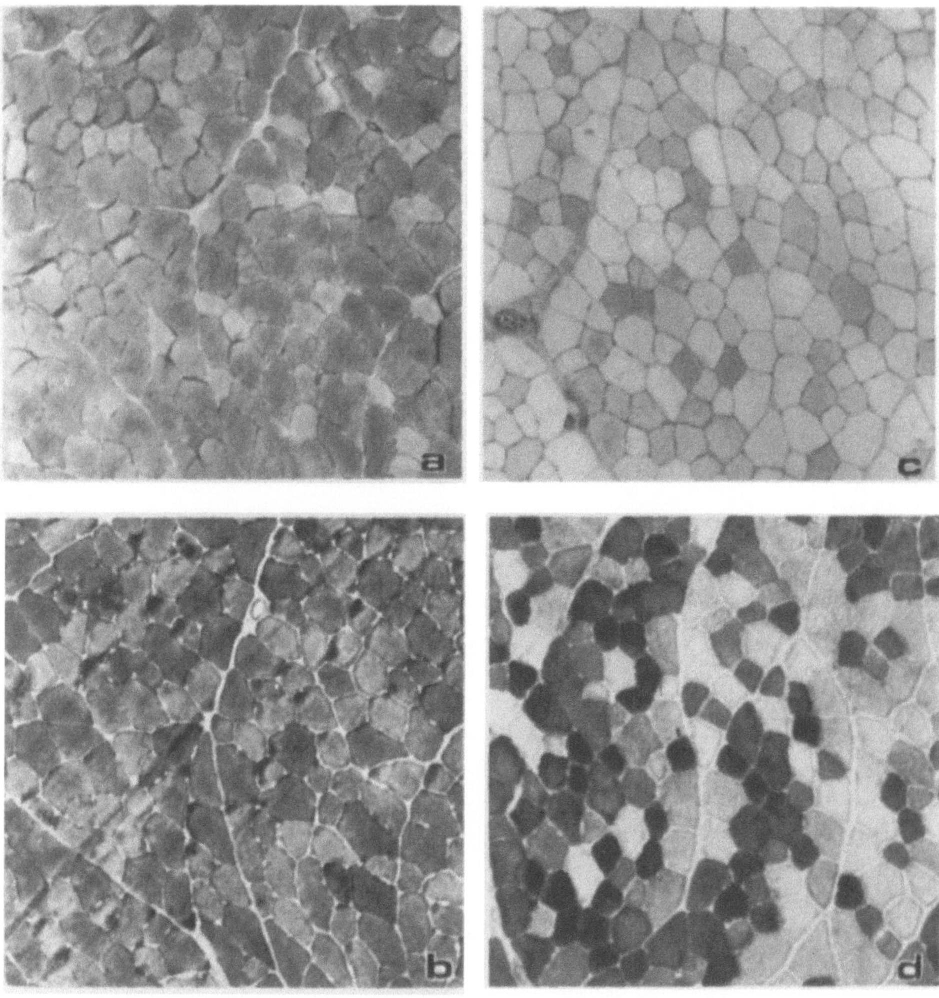

Fig. 5a-d. Tibialis anterior, deep layer, acute intoxication.
(a) and (b): control sections; (c) and (d): 1 h following i.p.
injection of 300 mg/kg 2,4-D. Higher magnification from Fig. 4d.
(a) and (c): PAS reaction for primary glycogen; (b) and (d):
phosphorylase reaction. Selective decrease in glycogen and in
phosphorylase (c) and (d) in $2B/A_m$ fibres, increase in $2A/C_m$
fibres. See also Fig. 6. Detail from section on which the counts
of Table 4 were performed. x 112

In the interpretation of these results reference is made prin-
cipally to the findings in the anterior tibial muscle. These
indicate that at the time of excision the superficial and mid-
layers of muscle can retain phosphorylase, whereas there is an
efflux of enzyme and glycogen from the deep region (Fig. 4).
Consequently, the histochemical enzyme reaction, proceeding
in three dimensions in the gelatin film but in only two in the
section, induces in the latter a condition of relative substrate
(G1P) deficiency, which is reflected in decreased formation of

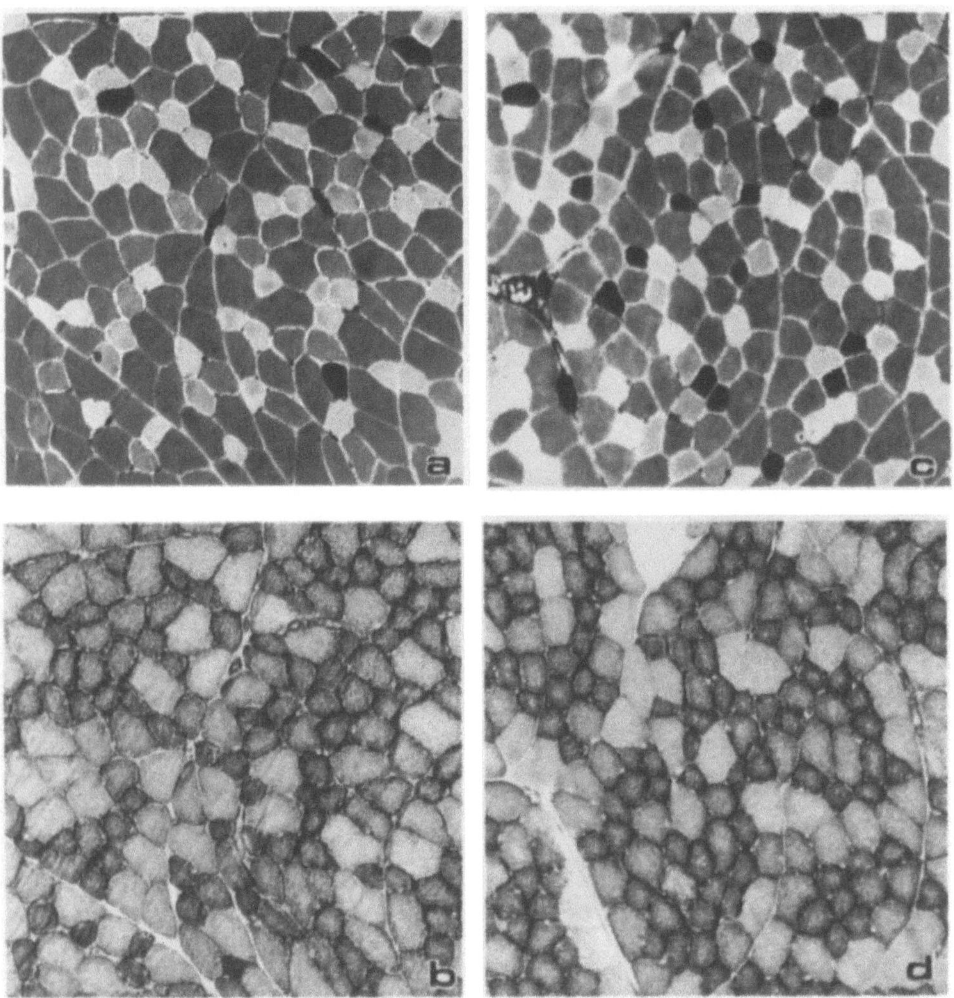

Fig. 6a-d. Tibialis anterior, serial to Fig. 5 for demonstration of fibre types. (a) and (c): ATPase, preincubated at pH 4.6; (b) and (d): NADH-TR. Corresponding fibre-type composition in sections from controls and from experimental animals. Opposite to findings from Fig. 5 (phosphorylase and glycogen), no changes can be observed in histochemical enzyme activities (ATPase, NADH-TR). x 112

amylopectin. Thus, the lowered substrate concentration, which develops in the vicinity of the section during incubation, may be expected to limit the formation of amylopectin more effectively in the section than in the gelatin film. The reciprocal activities of the enzyme in the section and in its gelatin film, in particular in the deep layers of muscle, can be explained by these factors. Since the proportion of "activated" $2A/C_m$ fibres deep within the muscle is small (12.6% of the cells of this region), the efflux of phosphorylase from these cells cannot

Table 4. Phosphorylase activity and glycogen content of the deep layer of
the anterior tibial muscle. Results taken from Fig. 5

| Fibre type | Phosphorylase Activity | | | Staining for |
ATP/mitoch. % of total fibre count (n = 357)	low or zero	medium or "normal"	increased	Primary Glycogen
$2A/C_m$ (32.2)	21.6 / /	/ 49.6 /	/ / 28.8^b	negative low to medium increased
$2B/A_m$ (60.8)	47.0 / /	/ 47.5 /	/ / $5.5^{a,b}$	negative low to medium increased
$1/B_m$ (7.0)	40.0 /	/ 60	/ /	low medium

Bracketed numbers indicate % of total fibre population (n = 357), other
numbers indicate % of the respective fibre types.

[a] mitochondrial content is higher than in typical A_m fibres.

[b] brownish amylopectin.

account for the total amount of amylopectin synthesized in the
incubation film. Furthermore, it is improbable that the reciprocal staining intensities in the section and in the film result from topically different states of activation of the enzyme,
though this cannot be entirely excluded. Essentially, the findings in the anterior tibial muscle indicate that an overall decrease in phosphorylase activity of the sections is brought
about by 2,4-D. An efflux of enzyme from the muscle cell, and
in particular from the white $2B/A_m$ fibres, ensues from the
action of this substance in vivo. As indicated by the findings
in the triceps surae and anterior tibial muscles, the time
course of efflux of the enzyme evidently differs in different
muscles as well as in different layers of a given muscle. At
present we cannot say whether these histochemical changes are
due to direct or to indirect action of 2,4-D. Since the experimental animals had been more or less immobilized by the
intoxication, the observed histochemical alterations, particularly those in the $2B/A_m$ fibres, are unlikely to be due to
differences in the mechanical and metabolic activity of the
various motor units (51, 89, 181).

As concerns the observed increase in phosphorylase activity in
a proportion of $2A/C_m$ fibres, histochemistry can only provide
limited evidence toward its interpretation. The $2A/C_m$ and the
sparse $2B/A_m$ fibres involved in this change differ from the
bulk of fibres of these types in their increased amounts of
primary glycogen and of NADH-TR activity. Hence, these fibres
display the criteria of both aerobic and anaerobic metabolism
(247). Biochemically, HØSTMARK and HORN (156) observed cor-

responding alterations in the diaphragm of rats. They showed
that fluoro- and iodo-acetate, which inhibit glycerin-3-phos-
phate dehydrogenase, can effect activation of cAMP-dependent
phosphorylase.[3] The authors suggested that the mechanism underlying these changes might be activation of phosphorylase-kinase
by means of an increase in free intracellular calcium ions, the
amount needed being estimated to be inferior to that eliciting
contraction. Hence, the changes in phosphorylase activity must
be regarded as secondary phenomena. The findings of KUHN and
STEIN (184) provide indirect evidence of comparable effects
of 2,4-D on the metabolism of muscle fibres. According to these
authors, 2,4-D delays the uptake of calcium into the vesicles
of the sarcoplasmic reticulum. Recent biochemical investigations
(136, 144, 209) have revealed the close molecular relationship
between calcium efflux from the sarcoplasmic vesicles, activation
of phosphorylase, and cleavage of ATP in muscular contraction.

C. Histological and Histochemical Findings in the Myopathy of Subacute Intoxication with 2,4-D (svi)

I. Skeletal Muscle (Triceps Surae)

1. Changes in the Developing Disease

a) Early Stage

In the early stage of the disease, e.g. on the 6th day of treatment, sections from the gastrocnemius muscle display different
degrees of involvement in different fibre types. The earliest
and severest alterations in the course of the disease are observed in the superficial layer of this muscle, consisting predominantly of $2B/A_m$ fibres (Figs. 7 and 8). With increasing
proportions of $1/B_m$ (intermediate) and $2A/C_m$ (red) fibres in
the deeper layers of the muscle, 2 B/A_m (white) fibres are subject to less marked changes as compared to the superficial
region. From observations with the light microscope, both
$1/B_m$ and $2A/C_m$ fibres are apparently unaltered in any layer
of the muscle. No changes can be detected in the soleus muscle.

A typical pattern of cytological dedifferentiation of white
$(2B/A_m)$ fibres can be demonstrated in the early stage of the
disease (Fig. 8). With the modified trichrome stain and, more
distinctly with the reactions for SDH and menadione-dependent
GDH, the perimyofibrillar pattern of these cells appears ir-
regular, rarefied and granular. In more advanced stages only
dash-shaped spots of activity can be seen, distributed over
the whole cross-section of the fibres. Compared to controls,

---

[3]It is remarkable that these authors, too, could not demonstrate
any inhibition of glycogen synthetase.

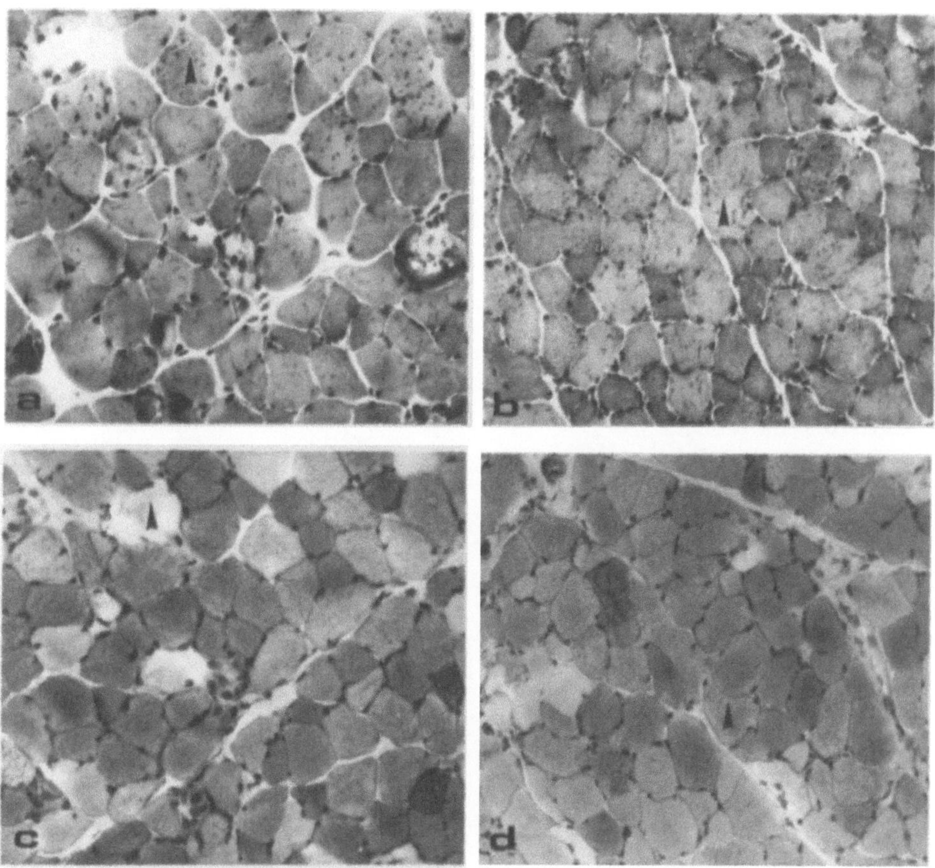

Fig. 7a-d. Gastrocnemius, subacute intoxication (svi), serial
sections, advanced stage of myopathy. (a) and (b): trichrome;
(c) and (d): primary glycogen (PAS-hematoxylin). Marked alterations and numerous necroses in the superficial (a) and (c) as
opposed to the deep (b) and (d) layers of the muscle. ▲ indicates
identical cell in (a) and (c), and in (b) and (d). x 112

the SDH pattern of the diseased fibres appears sparse and ir-
regular with marked activity in the subsarcolemmal space. The
fibre square-sections are not enlarged, indicating that swelling
does not occur at this stage. The nuclei are normal in size and
shape and are lying in a normal, subsarcolemmal position. In
longitudinal sections the cross-striation of muscle fibres can
be clearly observed. The muscle fibres are prone throughout
their length to intermyofibrillar disorganization.

The overall histochemical activity of the NAD- and NADP-dependent dehydrogenases (diaphorases), demonstrated as lactate dehydrogenase and as glucose-6-phosphate dehydrogenase, appear
unchanged as against the controls. The same is true of phosphorylase and glycogen synthetase activities and glycogen content.
Within this pattern, single $2B/A_m$ fibres in some regions display

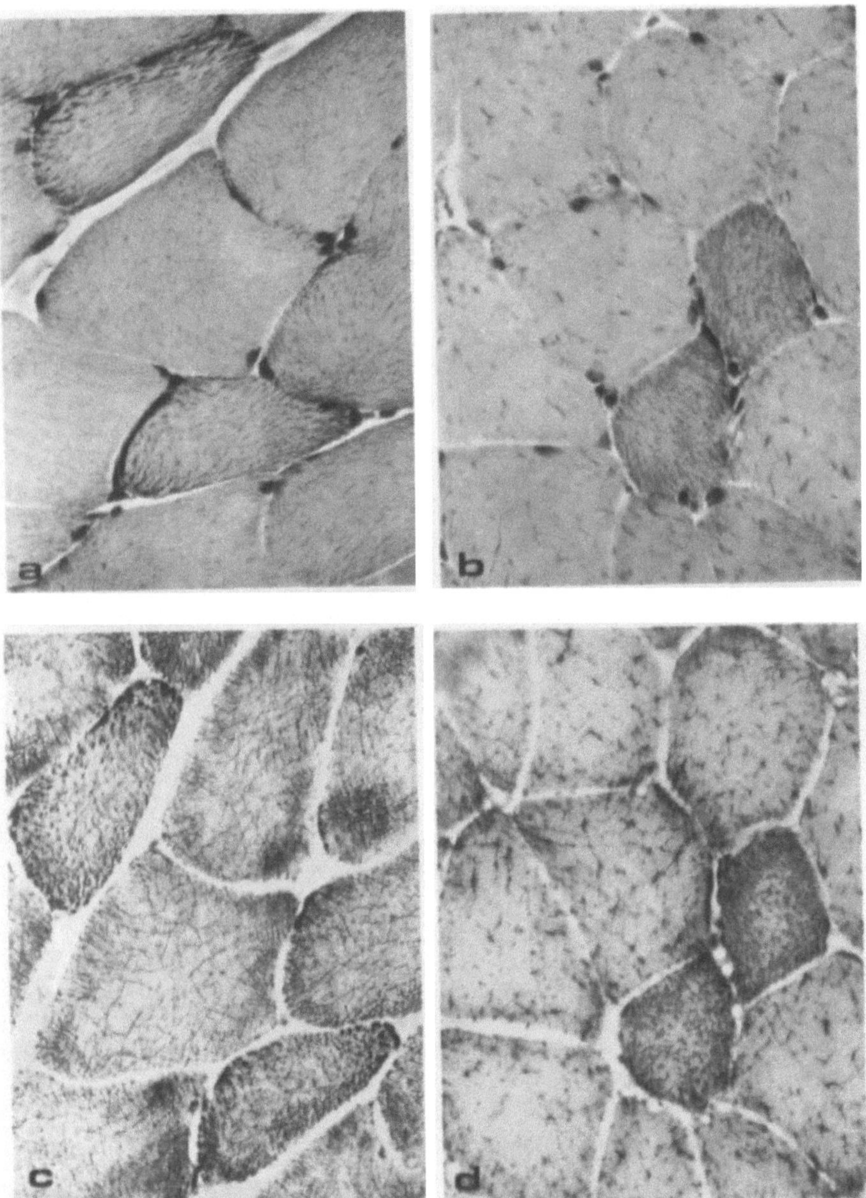

Fig. 8a-d. Gastrocnemius (svi), early stage of myopathy. (a) and
(c): control sections; (b) and (d): incipient myopathy. Upper:
trichrome, lower: menadione-GDH. Rarefied, granular perimyofibrillar reaction pattern of $2B/A_m$ fibres in (b) and (d). $2A/C_m$ fibres
unchanged. x 450

a decrease in glycogen and phosphorylase activity, the activity
of glycogen synthetase being increased in parallel. The SDH- and
menadione-linked GDH reactions of these fibres display the type
of incipient alterations described above (Fig. 9). Some scattered
fibres, not differing in phosphorylase activity from normal white

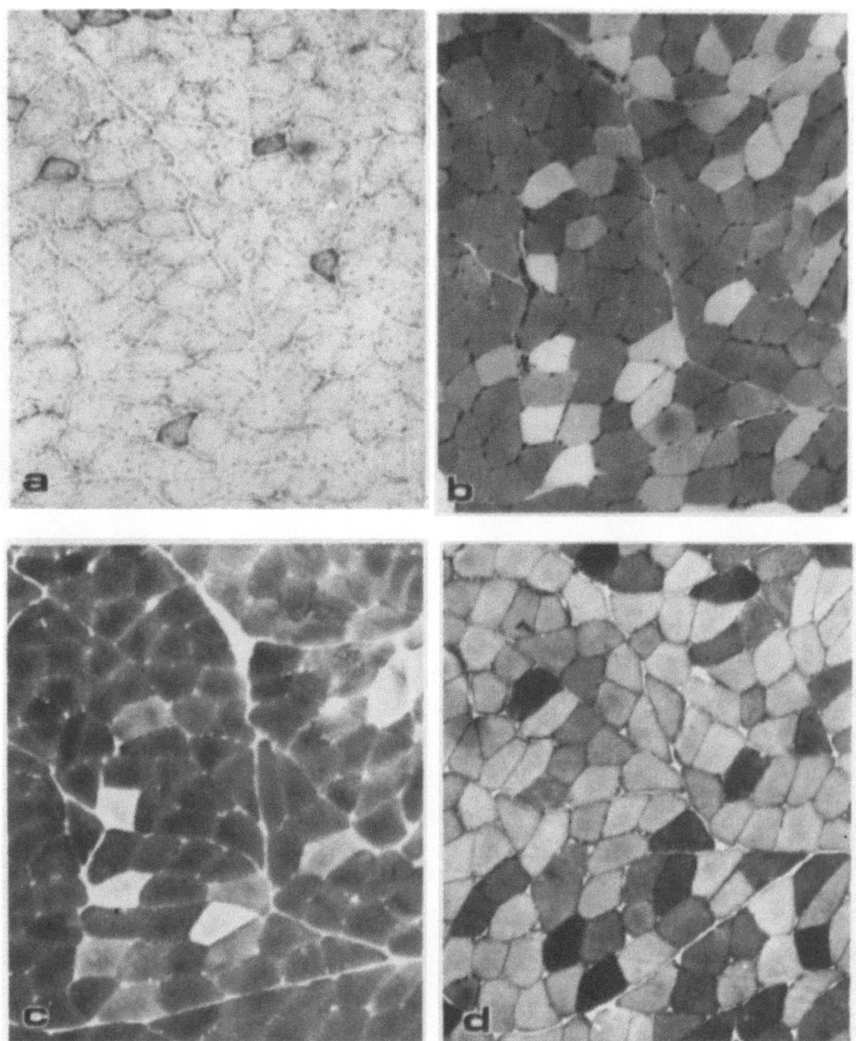

Fig. 9a-d. Gastrocnemius (svi), serial sections, early stage of myopathy. (a): SDH; (b): glycogen; (c): phosphorylase; (d): UDPG-GS. Cytological alterations corresponding to those in Fig. 8d. Decrease in glycogen and in phosphorylase in single $2B/A_m$ fibres, UDPG-GS activity being retained. x 112

$2B/A_m$ fibres, show much increased levels of glycogen synthetase. As concluded from the phosphorylase reaction of the entire section, an overall decrease in phosphorylase and glycogen synthetase activities preceding the initial cytological alterations of white muscle fibres ($2B/A_m$) cannot be demonstrated histochemically at this stage of the disease process. The myosin-ATPase reaction, which is unchanged, proves that the 2B-type of muscle fibre will be predominantly involved in these changes.

More severe alterations of single muscle fibres can already be observed at the initial stage of the disease, such as segmental

swelling and incipient vacuolization of white fibres (Figs. 10
and 11). The sarcoplasm yields a less intense staining. Nuclei,
lying in a subsarcolemmal position, are slightly enlarged. As
argued from the menadione-dependent GDH reaction, the cytological pattern of swollen fibres resembles that of unswollen ones
at the stage of intermyofibrillar dedifferentiation. In contrast
to this, the SDH reaction of swollen fibres is negative, the
reactivities for phosphorylase and for glycogen being also markedly reduced or negative (Fig. 10). The myofibrillar pattern of
such fibres appears thickened and their cross-striation blurred.
Dehydrogenase reactions other than that of SDH do not, however,

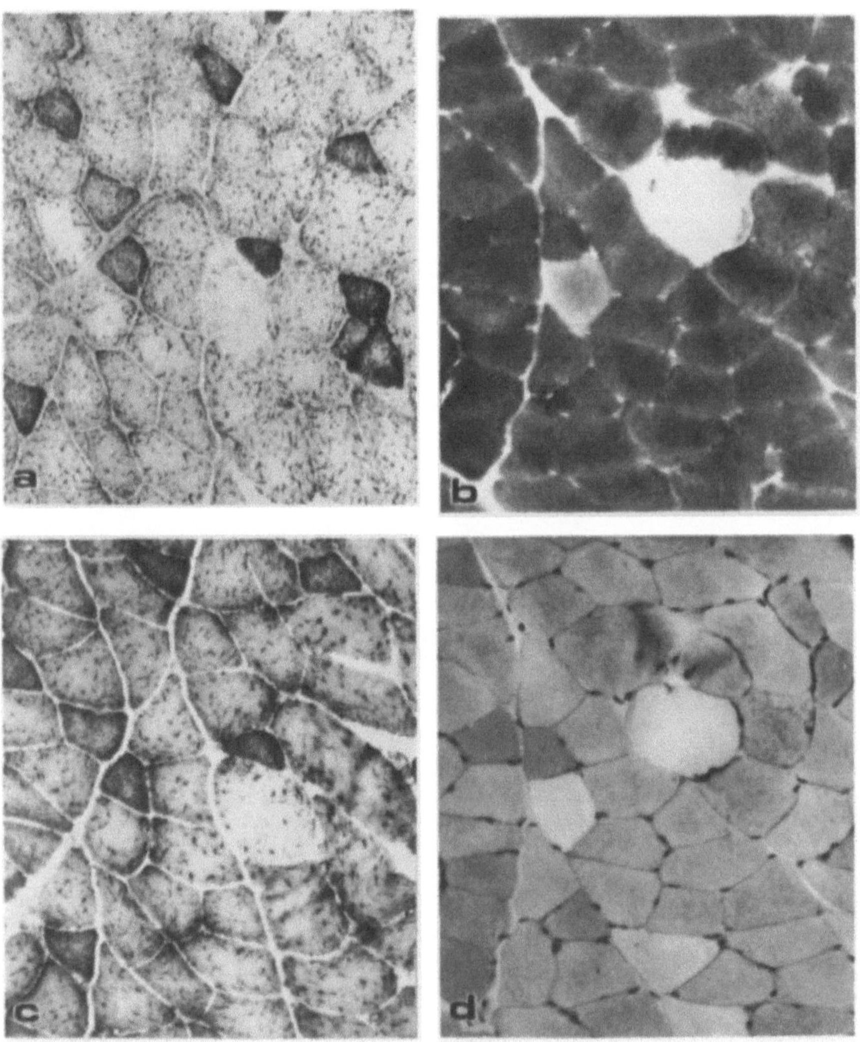

Fig. 10a-d. Gastrocnemius (svi), serial sections, early stage
of myopathy. Single swollen fibre with loss of SDH (a), phosphorylase activity (b) and glycogen (d). Menadione-GDH pattern
(c) relatively unchanged. x 180

allow any distinction to be made between swollen fibres and unswollen ones at the stage of intermyofibrillar disorganization.
Again, the ATPase type-2 fibres are the only ones involved in
swelling.

The histochemical findings described above strongly suggest that
alterations in mitochondria, mitochondrial enzyme activities
and glycogen metabolism occur immediately prior to the earliest
histological changes of the muscle fibre in this myopathy. Fine
clefts in the sarcoplasm of swollen fibres are the first signs
of vacuolization. As the disease advances, these vacuoles en-
large (Fig. 11). Fibre necrosis can also be observed without
preceding vacuolization: The sarcoplasm shows an increase in
eosinophilia and the interstitial cells are increased in number
with enlargement of their nuclei. Since, overall, fibre swelling
is rather a rare event, it is unlikely to constitute an obligatory transitional stage toward necrosis. In necrotic stages the
histochemical determination of fibre types can no longer be performed, so the type of fibres involved must be evaluated by
means of the preferential fibre type and of the types of fibres
which are uninvolved in the respective area. It can be stated
that $1/B_m$ and $2A/C_m$ fibres, both rich in mitochondria, display
none or only minor alterations in the form of disorganization
of the intermyofibrillar pattern.

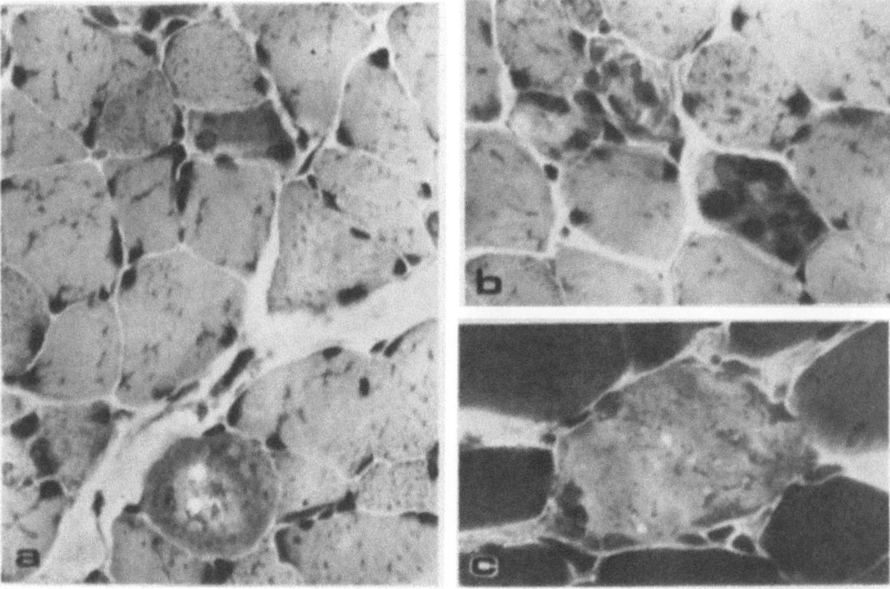

Fig. 11a-c. Gastrocnemius (svi), advanced stage of myopathy,
trichrome. Different stages of necrosis of muscle fibres. (a):
swelling with vacuolar degeneration; (b): necrosis with cellular reaction; (c): incipient stage of vacuolar degeneration.
(a) and (b): x 280; (c): x 450

b) Full Stage

The <u>full stage</u> of the disease process, as reached after 13 days
of continued treatment, shows different degrees of involvement
of 2B/A_m fibres, including states from fibre swelling to necrosis. Interposed C_m and B_m fibres actually appear uninvolved
(see Fig. 7). The severest alterations of 2B/A_m fibres occur
in the superficial layers of the gastrocnemius muscle, where
this fibre type prevails. The smallest degree of change in

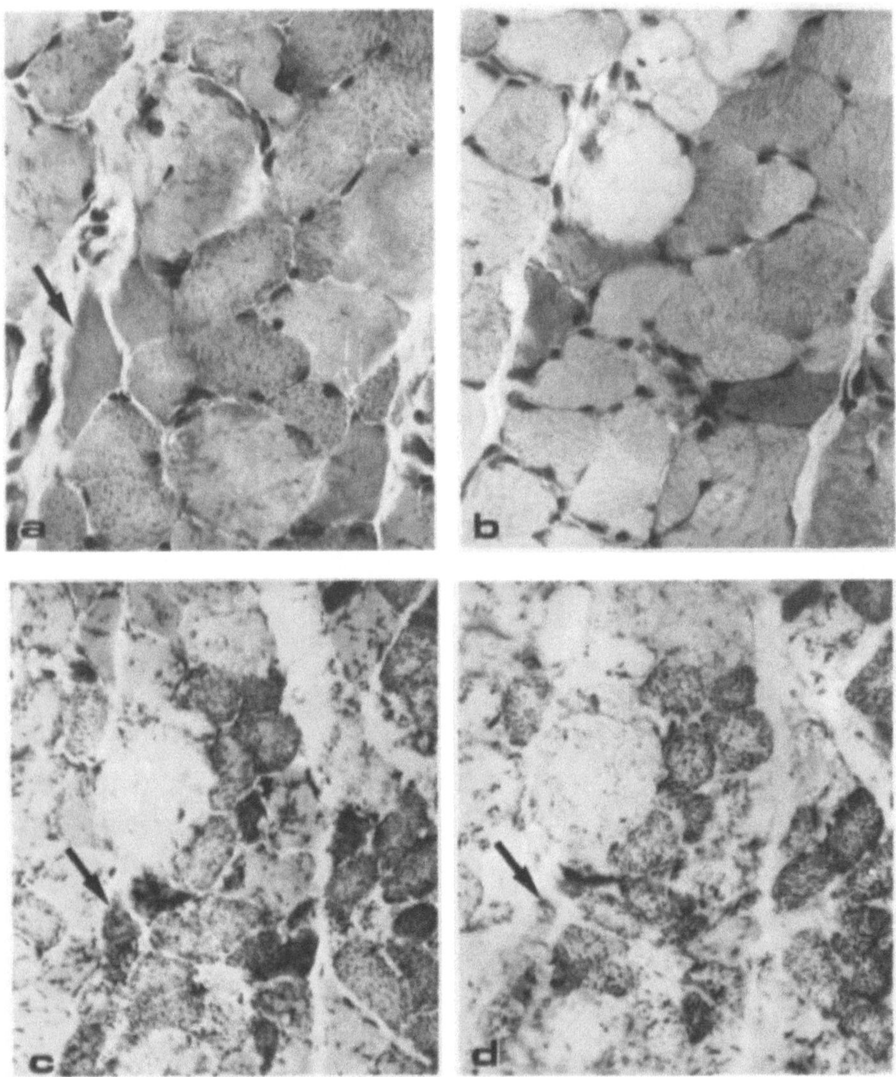

<u>Fig. 12a-d.</u> Gastrocnemius, advanced stage of myopathy. Atrophic
fibres (⟶) as well as myopathic fibres. (a): trichrome; (b):
glycogen; (c): NADH-TR; (d): SDH. Glycogen content of atrophic
fibres is increased (b); note positive NADH-TR (c) and negative
SDH reactions (d). Serial sections. (a) and (b): x 450; (c) and
(d): x 280

these fibres corresponds exactly with the stage of intermyofibrillar disorganization. Numerous swollen fibres with a darkly staining sarcoplasm can be observed in the vicinity of necrotic muscle fibres (Figs. 11 and 12).

Histochemical reactions indicate a pronounced overall decrease in glycolytic and oxidative enzyme activities. Residual activities of a granular appearance, suggestive of oxidative enzymes, are partly due to macrophages. Depending upon the degree of fibre damage, individual fibres can completely fail to show residual activities. Swelling, and the succeeding stages of fibre deterioration, are accompanied by negative reactions for glycogen and phosphorylase as well as for glycogen synthetase (Fig. 12).

Besides these myopathic changes, another type of alteration can be observed in advanced stages of the disease. Small, irregularly shaped angular fibres with densely staining sarcoplasm (Fig. 12) are interspersed between muscle fibres at varying stages

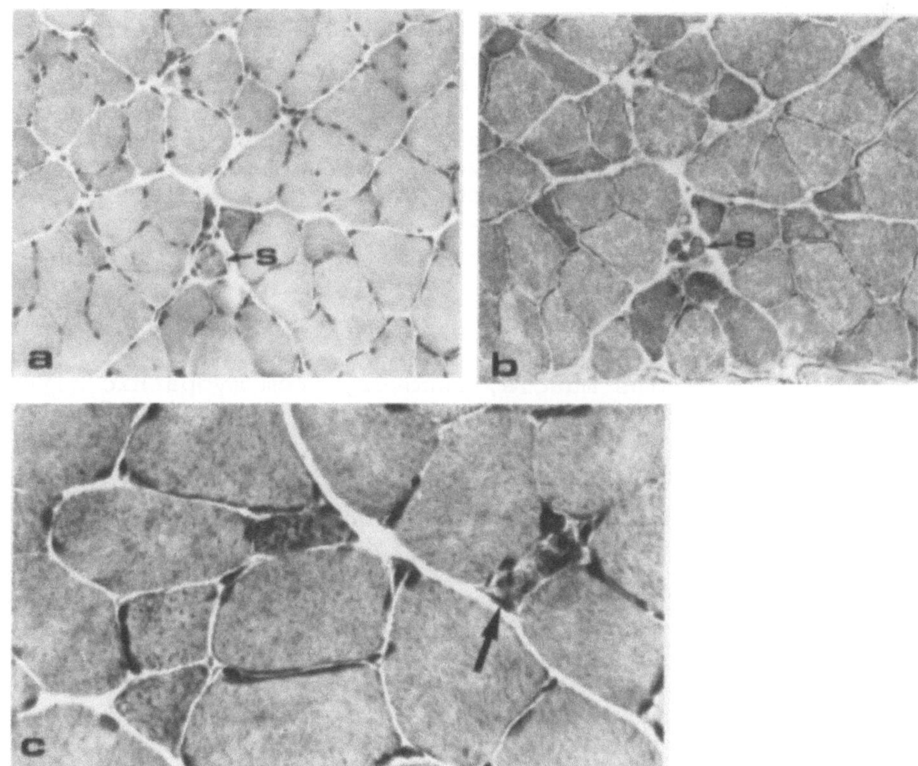

Fig. 13a-c. Soleus (svi), advanced stage of myopathy. Same animal as for Fig. 7. (a) and (c): trichrome; (b): SDH. Unchanged cytological pattern in (a) and (b); single necrosis of 2A/C_m fibres in (c) ($\longrightarrow$). S: muscle spindle. (a) and (b): x 180, (c): x 450

of necrosis. These angular fibres show up as type-1 or type-2, but the fibre type cannot always be clearly assessed from the ATPase reaction. Their occurrence is limited to areas where $2B/A_m$ fibres predominate, i.e. to the superficial and mid-layers of the muscle, whereas they cannot be found in the deep layers, or in the soleus muscle. As suggested by these topical relationships and the fact that these fibres yield a blue-violet iodine stain for phosphorylase activity, they may be assumed to correspond to white ($2B/A_m$) muscle fibres. This suggestion is further supported by observations during regeneration of these cells. Histologically they are most likely to be atrophic fibres. Unlike myopathic fibres, they are not prone to segmental degeneration but show atrophy along the whole of their length, as seen in serial sections. There is no increase in the number of nuclei. The nuclei are slightly enlarged and only exceptionally situated in central parts of the fibre. Glycogen is present in different and even increased amounts. The SDH reaction of the atrophic fibres if completely negative, whereas the NAD-dependent dehydrogenases show residual activities, yielding a homogeneous staining of the whole fibre cross-section.

In striking contrast to the severe involvement of the gastrocnemius is that of the soleus muscle (Fig. 13). The predominating type of large $1/B_m$ fibres in this muscle is completely spared by the disease process. As demonstrated by the LDH reaction, the cytological structure of the small $2A/C_m$ fibres remains intact or is only slightly altered. The glycogen content is decreased. Rare fibres of this type display simple necrosis. Alterations corresponding to those observed in $2B/A_m$ fibres of the gastrocnemius muscle are not seen in the course of the disease.

2. Changes during Recovery

In the gastrocnemius muscle, recovery from myopathic alterations can be distinguished from atrophic ones. Remission from myopathic changes proceeds faster. The number of internal nuclei is increased during regeneration. Eleven days after the end of treatment, fibre necrosis is no longer observed. In serial sections segmental differences of regeneration in individual muscle fibres can be seen. Segments displaying a fully reorganized perimyofibrillar network and nuclei in a subsarcolemmal position alternate with segments showing increased and enlarged internal nuclei. The sarcoplasm presents normal staining qualities. Internal nuclei can still be observed in fully reorganized fibres. By means of dehydrogenase reactions, targetoid fibres can be demonstrated to be at intermittent stages of regeneration, the central parts of some muscle fibres being still not fully reorganized (Fig. 14). In single muscle fibres with enlarged cross-sections and with a centrally placed large nucleus, septa continuous with the sarcolemma can be observed. Groups of thin muscle fibres of the ATPase type 2 can be seen in the surroundings of these elements (Fig. 15). This kind of change can be regarded as evidence of numerical regeneration by longitudinal fibre division.

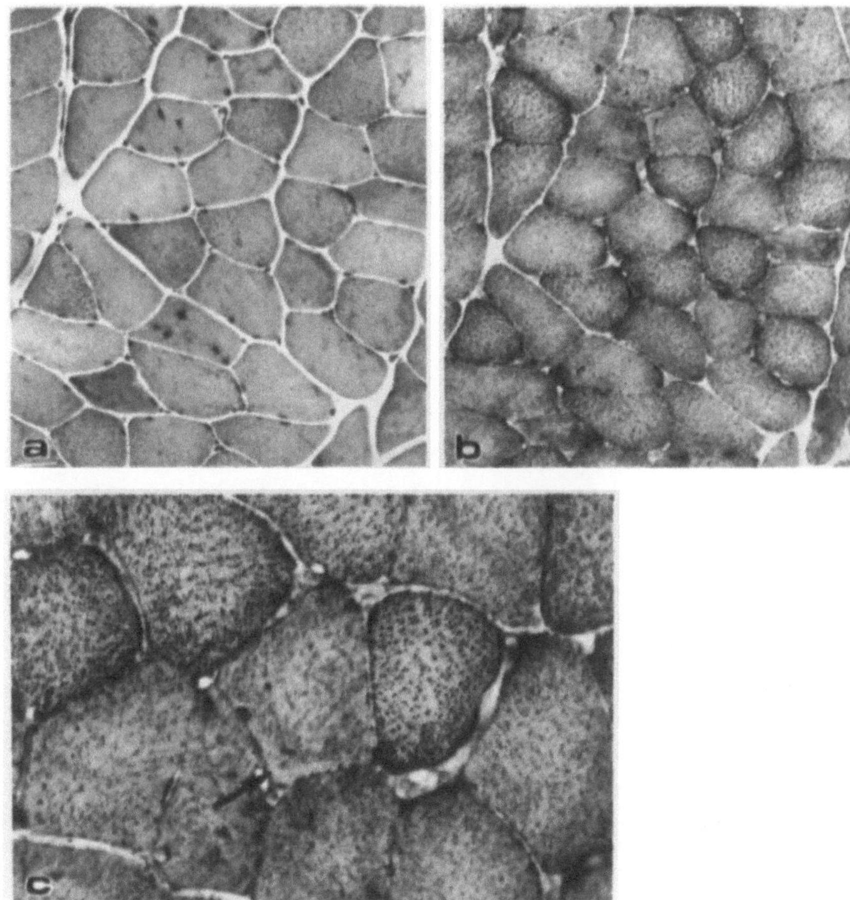

Fig. 14a-c. Gastrocnemius (svi), remission of myopathic changes.
(a): trichrome; (b) and (c): menadione-GDH. Increase in number
of central nuclei (a), distinct structure of marginal layers as
compared to blurred appearance of central parts of single fibres
(⟶) in (c). (a) and (b): x 180; (c): x 450

The regeneration of atrophic fibres gives rise to the appearance
of concavely shaped, angular muscle cells (Fig. 16). Histological staining reveals two concentric zones within these fibres;
a densely staining marginal zone and a brightly staining central
zone. As concluded from the positive ATPase reaction of the
reorganized marginal layer, these cells are type-2 fibres. The
reactions for glycogen, phosphorylase and glycogen synthetase
are positive in the marginal zone as well (Fig. 16). The nuclei
are not enlarged and are situated in the subsarcolemmal space.
By means of the menadione-dependent GDH reaction a blurred
internal structure can be disclosed in these cells. The activities of oxidative enzymes are highest in the marginal layer.
As observed in the severe stage of the disease process, the
SDH reaction of the atrophic cells is lower than in intact
fibres, including regenerated myopathic fibres. Recovery from
atrophy proceeds at different speeds in different segments of
the fibres (Fig. 16).

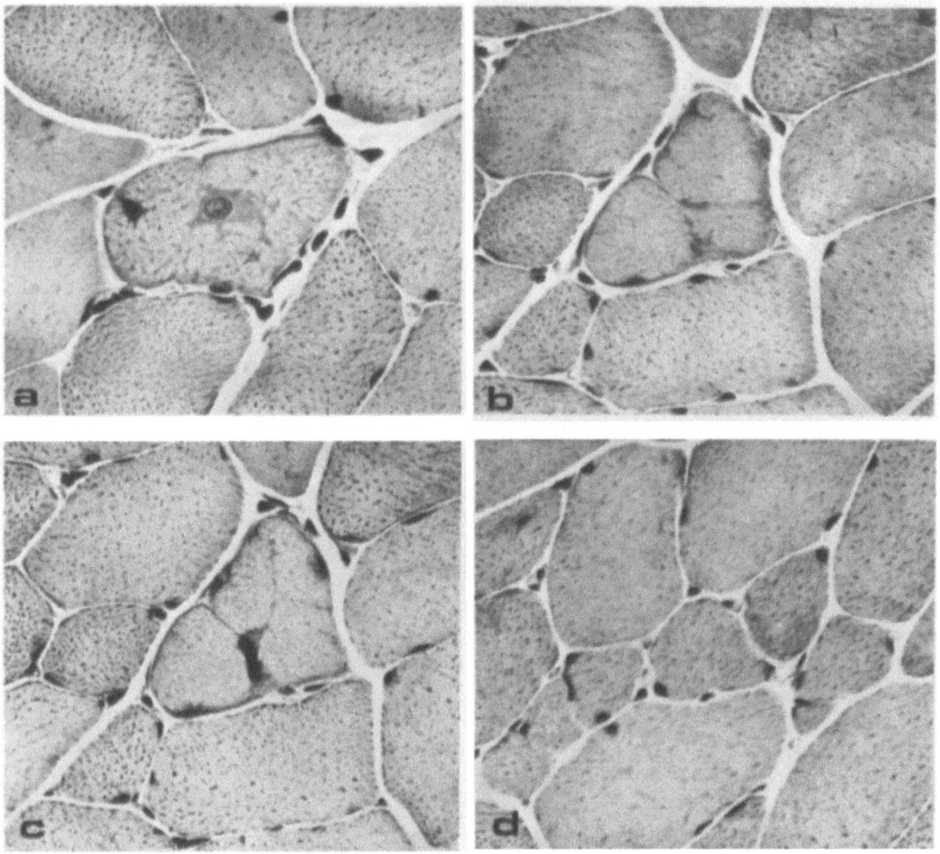

Fig. 15a-d. Gastrocnemius (svi), trichrome. Remission of myopathic changes. (a), (b) and (c): serial sections. Different
stages of longitudinal fibre division with centrally situated
myoblast nucleus (a). (d): cluster of thin muscle fibres resulting from longitudinal division of a parent fibre. x 450

Histochemically, the atrophic fibres differ from the myopathic
ones in their glycogen content and phosphorylase activity. In
the developing disease, the atrophic fibres display varying
and mostly raised levels of glycogen and of phosphorylase.
Both these constituents also yield increased staining during
recovery. In contrast, myopathic fibres that have passed the
stage of fibre swelling are depleted of glycogen and negative
for phosphorylase and glycogen synthetase activities. The
muscle fibres of the soleus during recovery do not show any
clear structural alterations. In the red $2A/C_m$ fibres numerous
lipid droplets can be observed all over the fibre cross-section.
Staining for glycogen, for phosphorylase and for glycogen
synthetase activities in the soleus muscle of treated animals
does not differ from that of controls.

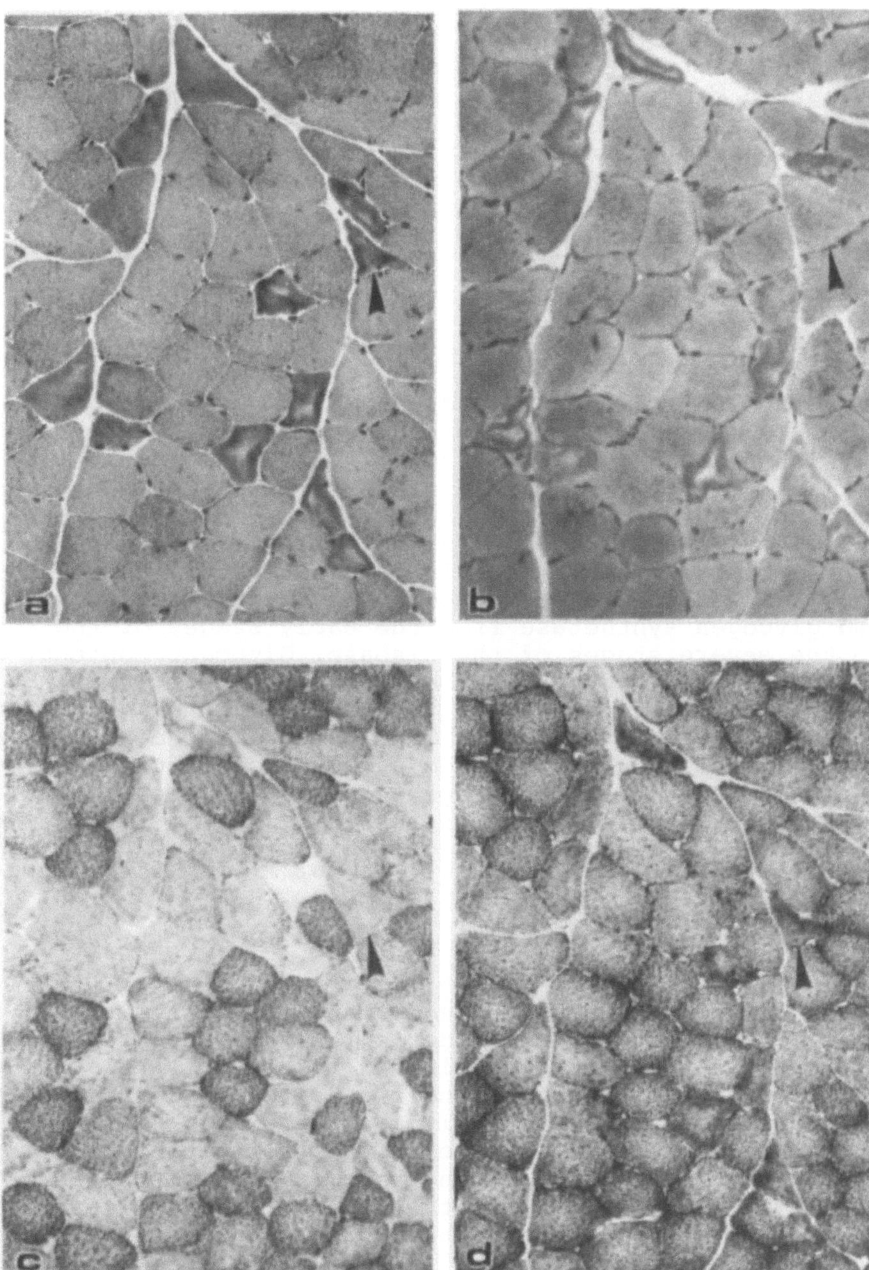

Fig. 16.a-d. Gastrocnemius (svi), serial sections. Remission of atrophic changes. (a): trichrome; (b): glycogen; (c): SDH; (d): menadione-GDH. Targetoid structure of atrophic fibres (a) with negative SDH stain (c). Segmental differences in regeneration of individual fibres (►). x 180

Over the experimental period, no increase could be demonstrated
in the amount of connective tissue and number of fat cells in
the superficial layers of the gastrocnemius muscle, where the
myopathic changes were most outstanding. From the severe stage
of the disease to incipient regeneration there was an increase
in the number of interstitial histiocytes. No evidence could
be obtained at the light-microscopic level of involvement of
the blood vessels and myelinated nerve fibres in these experiments.

II.   Myocardium of the Ventricles

Histochemically, the myocardium of the ventricles in the rat
consists of $2C/C_m$ fibres, yielding a strong ATPase reaction
within the range pH 9.4 to 4.3. In skeletal muscle of adult
animals this type of muscle fibre is rarely encountered. In
contrast to the changes in skeletal muscle, during the entire
course of this myopathy no histological alterations could be
demonstrated in the myocardium of the ventricles. A decline
was observed in the histochemical activities of phosphorylase
and glycogen synthetase from the early stages of the myopathy
to the severe stages of the disease. Glycogen content, which
histochemically appears to be low in the heart, was not actually changed in the course of the disease. Other enzyme activities, in particular that of SDH, were histochemically unchanged.
Alterations in cardiac rhythm suggesting conduction block could
be observed outlasting decapitation of the experimental animals.
Histological and histochemical studies were not performed as
regards these findings.

III.   Liver

A depletion of glycogen, predominantly from the portal areas of
the liver lobule, occurred during the disease process. This depletion was present in the initial stages of the subacute myopathy of 2,4-D as well as under conditions of acute intoxication.
In advanced stages of the disease there was extensive loss of
glycogen proceeding from the portal to the central parts of the
liver lobule (Fig. 17). When treatment was discontinued, remission of the alterations of the liver proceeded faster than that
of the myopathic changes. The decrease in histochemical phosphorylase activity occurred in parallel with glycogen depletion
of the liver. In the severest stages of the disease, the phosphorylase activity was absent in the liver. During recovery,
the lowered activity of this enzyme outlasted the fall in glycogen content. No changes were seen in the activity of glycogen
synthetase in the liver. Staining with methyl green-pyronine
gave no evidence of interference with RNA synthesis in the liver
cell. The oil-red-O stain revealed a marked increase in the
number of fat droplets, especially in liver cells of the portal
area. At the height of the myopathy the activities of NAD- and
NADP-dependent dehydrogenases of the liver were depressed, as

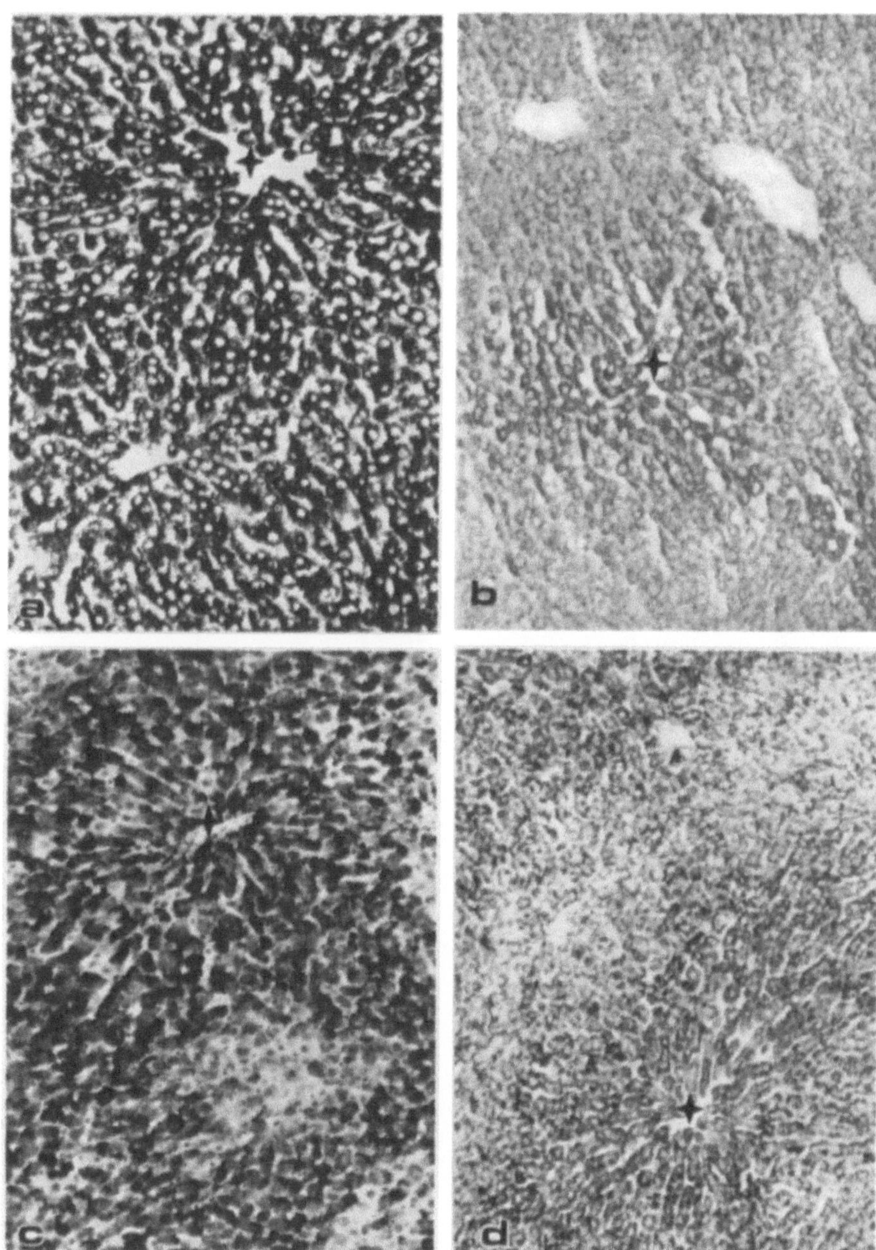

Fig. 17a-d. Liver (svi). (a) and (c): controls; (b) and (d): advanced stages of the myopathy. (a) and (b): G-6-PDH; (c) and (d): primary glycogen; marked decrease, accentuated in the periphery of the liver lobule, of G-6-PDH activity and glycogen content in the experimental animals. Asterisk: central vein. x 112

was clearly demonstrated by the G-6-PDH reaction (Fig. 17). The activity of SDH, on the contrary, did not appear to be altered. During recovery, lowered activities of menadione-dependent GDH activity lasted longer than the decrease in the activities of other dehydrogenases. The typical dehydrogenase pattern of the liver lobule was not altered by the disease process. Thus, in the case of the NADP-dependent dehydrogenases (G-6-PDH), enzyme loss was most marked from areas of lowest primary activities, i.e. the periphery of the liver lobule (Fig. 17). This refers to enzyme activities as displayed by the homogeneous, non-granular cytoplasmic formazan staining of the liver cells. In addition, granular formazan could be observed in the sinus at the periphery of the liver lobules. The sinuoidal deposits together with weak intracellular staining reactions point to enzyme loss mainly from the portal areas.

Discussion and Conclusions

A. Muscle

Before the particular findings are discussed, an attempt, necessarily hypothetical, will be made to explain the alterations in skeletal muscle brought about by 2,4-D in both the acute and subacute intoxication experiments from the point of view of a common pathogenesis.

The histochemical findings in acute intoxication (avi) suggest that 2,4-D, like fluoro- and iodo-acetate, can act as an inhibitor of glycerin-3-phosphate dehydrogenase. This inhibition would induce compensatory activation of glycolysis (156) in red (2A/C_m; 1/B_m) muscle fibres but decompensatory cell damage in white fibres under conditions of lower aerobic yields and fully activated glycolysis, so giving rise to the efflux of enzyme and glycogen and the histological alterations observed in the experiments. Concomitantly, the sarcoplasmic reticulum to which glycogen and phosphorylase are bound (209) would be altered. The mitochondrial changes seen in 2B/A_m fibres in the early stage of subacute intoxication with 2,4-D (svi) could be interpreted as indicating a compensatory activation of aerobic metabolism. Histochemically, loss of phosphorylase activity would not be obligatory at this stage of cellular damage. Sparing of red and intermediate muscle fibres (2A/C_m, 1/B_m) would thus be due to the predominance of the aerobic energy supply with additional activation of glycolysis in these muscle cells. The findings presented here and in preceding studies (140, 141) suggest that there must be pathogenetic relationships like those described above which would link the changes seen in the acute myopathy of 2,4-D (avi) with those observed in the subacute variety of the disease process.

I. Early Stage of the Subacute Myopathy of 2,4-D

In seeking to make a pathogenetic evaluation of the findings in the myopathy of 2,4-D, one must consider the earliest changes occurring in skeletal muscle. Hence, this myopathy involves predilectively type-2 (2B/A_m) or white muscle fibres, whereas the myocardium of the ventricles is spared by the disease process.

The earliest alterations, as observed under the light microscope in sections stained for succinodehydrogenase, can be described as a disturbance of intermyofibrillar structure. This type of alteration was also observed in the myopathies induced by vincristine (56) and triamcinolone (49, 275), and in the hereditary dystrophy of the mouse (205).

The earliest lesions on the ultrastructural level were proliferative swelling and an increase in the number of mitochondria, accompanied or succeeded by swelling of the sarcoplasmic reticulum, as demonstrated in muscular dystrophy of the mouse (21, 240, 250, 269), in experimental corticosteroid myopathy (3, 49, 67, 68, 295, 296), in the myopathy of vitamin-E deficiency (299), in the myopathy of vincristine (56), in the acute myopathy of 2,4-D (142) and also in progressive muscular dystrophy of man (115). Hence, these alterations, which precede the myofibrillar lesions, are nonspecific (49, 115, 245, 298, 307).

In the subacute myopathy of 2,4-D, electron-microscopic studies have not yet been undertaken. The findings in other myopathies substantiate the conclusion that the earliest cytological alterations in the myopathy of 2,4-D, as seen under the light microscope, are paralleled at the ultrastructural level by nonspecific proliferation of mitochondria and of the sarcoplasmic reticulum of $2B/A_m$ fibres. Mitochondrial proliferation may be an adaptive response to the increased demands of oxidative metabolism. The sparing of red muscle fibres by the myopathic process can be interpreted as due to their higher oxidative capacities compared to white muscle fibres.

As regards the subsequent alterations, the findings in the myopathy of 2,4-D were similar to those in the myopathies of vincristine (56) and of triamcinolone (275), and indicated that the loss of glycogen and of phosphorylase activity from white muscle fibres immediately precedes or elicits the histological alterations, i.e. swelling and necrosis of the muscle fibre. Biochemically, a decrease in the activity of muscle phosphorylase was demonstrated in the early stages of different myopathies such as progressive muscular dystrophy of man (74, 75, 249, 261), myopathy of vitamin-E deficiency (190, 220), muscular dystrophy of the chicken (64) and hereditary dystrophy of the mouse (189, 257). Corresponding histochemical findings were described in hereditary dystrophy of the chicken and in corticosteroid myopathy of the rabbit (62, 63, 275, 276). However, a decrease in phosphorylase activity of skeletal muscle was also observed following denervation (158, 189).

The close connexion between altered glycolysis and histological fibre damage in the subacute myopathy of 2,4-D prompts the suggestion that the decrease in phosphorylase activity, detected biochemically in the myopathies cited above, is always due to different degrees of fibre necrosis. These findings clearly indicate that the decrease in phosphorylase activity in the various myopathies is unspecific. DREYFUS and SCHAPIRA (75) pointed out that in progressive muscular dystrophy of man a general decrease in the activities of glycolytic enzymes will be critically reflected in the activity of the enzyme that limits the rate of glycolysis. This enzyme is phosphorylase (75). In myogenesis, too, it is the activity of this enzyme which precedes and determines the development of other glycolytic enzyme activities (63).

The specific action of 2,4-D that initiates the unspecific histochemical and histological changes in unknown. Biochemical studies on rat skeletal muscle (182, 183) showed that in vitro 2,4-D can increase the concentrations of glycolytic metabolites and the uptake of oxygen. Since no corresponding histochemical experiments were performed, these findings cannot be interpreted in terms of fibre types. As mentioned above, these results could support the conclusion that 2,4-D causes inhibition of glycolysis in white ($2B/A_m$) fibres and compensatory activation of oxidative metabolism in red (C_m, B_m) fibres. It has been shown that the action of this substance in plants is to elicit a shift of metabolism from glycolysis towards oxidative glucose consumption by the pentose phosphate cycle (139, refs.). Furthermore, 2,4-D can influence the synthesis and uptake of RNA in the hypocotyl of the soya bean, thus inducing disturbed longitudinal growth (176, 245, refs.). A marked decrease in phosphorylase activity was observed in the stalk and leaves of red beans consequent to local treatment with 2,4-D (217). In cultured skeletal muscle cells, 2,4-D caused a reduction in DNA synthesis. Additional cytotoxic effects were also observed (242).

Whereas the early alterations of the intermyofibrillar structure are reversible after treatment is stopped, fibre swelling, once elicited, evidently proceeds to fibre necrosis.

II. Full Stage of the Subacute Myopathy of 2,4-D

At the histological level, the course run by the myopathy of 2,4-D is essentially similar to that of other primary myopathies (1). Following the segmental cloudy swelling of muscle fibres, (Zenker's) hyaline degeneration of the contractile substance can be observed, followed by histiocytic and phagocytic reactions and regenerative changes. This means that the discussion of the histological changes seen in the myopathy of 2,4-D can thus be restricted to particular aspects of the disease process.

It was claimed from findings concerning muscular dystrophy in the mouse (23) that hypertrophy of muscle fibres developed prior to swelling and dedifferentiation. This argument cannot be supported by the present findings which, on the contrary, indicate that fibre swelling and the later stages of fibre necrosis arise without preceding hypertrophy of the muscle fibre. Contrary to the conclusions of ERB (1891, cited in (234)), the same process has been shown to occur in progressive muscular dystrophy of man (101, 234).

The great variety of the degenerative changes seen in the later stages of the myopathy of 2,4-D indicates that, once elicited, the necrosis of muscle fibres can proceed at different rates, largely independently of any persistent effect of the agent. It is remarkable that necroses are more numerous in the superficial layers of the gastrocnemius muscle than in its deep layers, where relatively more $1/B_m$ and $2A/C_m$ fibres are present.

54

It has been well established by histological studies in warm-
blooded animals (61, 248) that capillarization is more extensive
in red than in white muscle. In physiological experiments in the
cat (147) resting blood flow measured in the soleus was four
times higher than in the gastrocnemius muscle. It can be assumed
that these differences correspond to differences in tissue oxygen
pressure. In man, it has been demonstrated (185) that the maximum
oxygen pressure is lower in myopathic than in normal muscle. It
has been concluded from this finding that simple hypoxic necrosis
of muscle fibres occurs in the course of myopathies (185). Similar
conclusions were reached on the basis of biochemical findings
concerning the binding of oxygen by myoglobin of muscle from
dystrophic chickens (9). The process of dystrophy was indeed decelerated by maintaining the animals at increased oxygen pres-
sures (10).

In the myopathy of 2,4-D the observation of minor changes in
white ($2B/A_m$) fibres of the deep layers of the gastrocnemius
muscle could thus be due to the "protective" effect of greater
capillarization and the correspondingly higher oxygen pressure
in these areas.

Special attention will be given to the occurrence of atrophic
fibres in the myopathy of 2,4-D. Similar observations were reported in chronic neuromyopathies (97). The atrophic fibres can
easily be distinguished from myopathic ones by their positive
reactions for glycogen and phosphorylase. The particular factors that give rise to neurogenic atrophy of scattered muscle
fibres in this myopathy are unknown. Since the atrophic fibres
are observed in areas where white muscle fibres predominate,
they are likely to belong to the same fibre type. Atrophy could
ensue through the involvement of their terminal axons by severe
myopathic alterations of neighbouring muscle fibres. The slower
recovery of the atrophic fibres also suggests possible transient
denervation. Since the atrophic fibres can only be observed in
later stages of the disease, they are likely to have been subject prior to denervation to the cytological alterations characteristic of the early stage of the myopathic process. This like-
lihood is further established by the negative SDH reaction of
the atrophic fibres in the full stage of the disease.

The absence of marked nuclear reactions in the atrophic fibres
may indicate that denervation takes place early in the disease
process. The reasons why atrophic fibres show no further myopathic changes are unknown. Apart from these findings, there
was no evidence over the experimental period of a general and
direct neurotoxic action of 2,4-D. It may well be suggested
that such effects are brought about by this substance as well
(187), but the preponderant involvement of skeletal muscle is
the main symptom of this intoxication.

The interference between myopathy and denervation of muscle was
studied in the muscular dystrophy of the mouse (23). Atrophy
of muscle fibres ensuing from severance of the sciatic nerve
was enhanced by the dystrophic process. In the myopathy of
vitamin-E deficiency in the rat, denervation or tenotomy slowed

down the appearance of myopathic changes, provided it was performed between the 5th and 17th day of life (227, 228). These
findings establish the decreased resistivity of dystrophic muscle fibres to denervation and the increased resistivity of
atrophic muscle fibres to the myopathic process. With some
critical reservations, they can partially apply to the atrophic
changes seen in the present myopathy.

Lesions of the terminal innervation, as suggested here, could
be displayed in the hereditary muscular dystrophy of the mouse
(133), in the myopathy of vitamin-E deficiency of the guinea
pig (55), and in Duchenne muscular dystrophy of man (165). In
the latter condition, only one out of 33 muscle biopsies showed
the terminal innervation to be apparently intact. Swelling and
collateral sprouting of subterminal axons was observed under the
light microscope. On the ultrastructural level there was almost
total absence of the functional folds, with swelling, shrinking
and fragmentation of the terminal expansions of the end-plates.
Electron-microscopic observations suggested that the "vitality"
of the neurone was not diminished. The changes seen were argued
to be secondary to primary disease of the muscle fibres (165).
In a recent study (167) no degeneration of nerve terminals or
of intramuscular nerve fibres was observed in Duchenne dystrophy.
The consistent abnormality was found to be focal atrophy of the
postsynaptic folds, which was associated with a significant decrease in the postsynaptic membrane profile concentration and
in the ratio of postsynaptic to presynaptic membrane length.
The study provided no morphological evidence for a diseased
motor neurone in Duchenne dystrophy, but it did not exclude,
as stated by the authors, any abnormal neural influence which
would not be reflected in a morphological alteration of the
motor nerve terminal. Neurophysiological studies dealing with
the possibility of a primary neurogenic alteration in Duchenne
muscular dystrophy can only be mentioned here (202, 203, 272).

III. Recovery Stage

Recovery of animals from the myopathy was almost complete within 10 days after stopping treatment. At this stage internal
nuclei could still be observed in some muscle fibres. The
prominence of the nucleolus and the basophilia of the perikaryon
suggested that some of these nuclei belonged to myoblasts.
Various stages of longitudinal fibre division could be observed,
as a sign of numerical regeneration of muscle fibres. This change
is known to occur in muscular dystrophy of man (ERB, cited by
(131)), in hypertrophy of normal muscle (DURANTE, cited by (131)),
in muscular dystrophy of the mouse (34), and in experimental hypertrophy of the soleus muscle in the rat (129).

From the present findings it can be concluded that a thorough
cytological restitution of the muscle cell, including the presence of internal nuclei, is a necessary condition of septation
and longitudinal fibre division (Fig. 13). The small fibres
emerging from this process display the same histological and
histochemical signs as the parent cell. By analogy with the ob-

servations in overloaded skeletal muscle of rats (130), longitudinal fibre division in the myopathy of 2,4-D can be interpreted
as ensuing from functional overload of the earliest regenerated
muscle fibres.

Regeneration of atrophic fibres gives rise to the appearance of
targetoid fibres (94, 99), as described in longstanding denervation processes. In these muscle cells an unstructured central
area consisting of disorganized myofilaments (264) is surrounded
by a marginal zone with preserved myofibrillar structure. In
2,4-D myopathy in particular, the targetoid fibres display
shrinkage and deformation of their shape, brought about by
neighbouring muscle fibres of normal appearance (96). The targetoid fibres are of the ATPase type 2, whereas their mitochondrial type cannot be strictly assessed.

B. Myocardium

As demonstrated in the experiments described, the ventricular
cardiac fibres of the rat present the same histochemical profile
as $2C/C_m$ fibres (38), which occur only rarely in the skeletal
muscle of adult animals. This type of fibre can be regarded as
representing a variety of red $1/C_m$ fibres, found in considerable
amounts in adult animals, which are closely related histochemically to the fibres of the ventricular myocardium. Further evidence
of this comes from biochemical findings in which the similarity
in the isozyme pattern of lactate dehydrogenase of the myocardium
and of red skeletal muscle has been established (290).

Our own experiments confirmed that the typological similarity
between the myocardium and $1/C_m$ fibres of the skeletal muscle
holds good for all stages of this myopathy. The high resistivity
of this type of fibres corresponds to the absence of any significant alteration in the myocardium at the light-microscopic
level. The observed decrease in phosphorylase activity in the
myocardium cannot, as an isolated change, be regarded under
present experimental conditions as indicative of a structural
change in the myocardium. Thus, at light-microscopic level, the
myopathy of 2,4-D shows another similarity to hereditary muscular
dystrophy of the mouse. Heterozygotes with focal degenerations
of skeletal muscle did not show any alteration of the heart (206).
In homozygotic animals with severe symptoms, the myocardium was
spared or involved only late in the disease process (164). In
addition, determinations of electrolyte content in diseased and
in control animals (317) revealed differences in skeletal, but
not in heart muscle.

Since the findings in the myopathy of 2,4-D apply only to the
ventricular myocardium, they cannot yield information as to
changes in the conduction system of the heart. The observed dissociation between atrial and ventricular contractions in the
diseased animals could be evidence of such alterations. It is
well established that the conduction system differs from the
myocardium in its histological properties and in its high glycogen content.

In contrast to the type of myopathy induced by 2,4-D, degeneration of red muscle fibres together with prominent alterations of the myocardium (192, 277) can be observed in the myopathy of chloroquine. Cardiomyopathy is an outstanding symptom of plasmocide intoxication (146), in which severe mitochondrial alterations (66, 303) and a decrease in the corresponding enzyme activities (19, 215, 303) have been found. The histological alterations consisted in vacuolization and colliquation necrosis of heart muscle fibres.

Summarizing, it can be concluded that primary involvement of the myocardium in the disease process is not to be expected in myopathies of type 2, in which the white fibres of skeletal muscle are predilectively altered.

C. Liver

Only a few studies have been concerned with the question of the involvement of the liver in experimental myopathies, but in muscular dystrophy of man this problem has been more closely considered (29, 145).

In muscular dystrophy of the mouse no differences could be detected in the creatine content of the liver as between diseased and control animals (172, refs.).

In the muscle of dystrophic animals 60% and 40% increases, respectively, in DNA and in RNA synthesis could be demonstrated by the use of radioactive glycine-^{14}C (57). Corresponding studies of the liver revealed no significant differences (57, 122), though the incorporation of glycine-^{14}C did decrease in proportion to the severity of the dystrophic process (57). It has been concluded from the results of studies of protein metabolism in the liver and skeletal muscle of the dystrophic mouse that the liver would not be involved in the disease process (273). In chloroquine myopathy (215) no histological alterations of the liver could be detected. Biochemically, no significant differences could be demonstrated in the activity of aldolase, succinodehydrogenase, cytochrome oxidase and cathepsine (309) in homogenates of the liver of dystrophic mice, nor could alterations in the activity of any of a series of NAD- and NADP-dependent dehydrogenases be ascertained. Some of these enzymes showed a tendency towards decreased activity (132).

The loss of glycogen and a concomitant decrease in the phosphorylase activity of the liver, already observed at early stages of the disease, as well as the diminished activities of NAD- and NADP-dependent dehydrogenases in the advanced stages, must be regarded as non-specific toxic effects of 2,4-D. These are accompanied by a reduction in body weight and a decline in the general condition of the animals. The toxic character of these alterations to the liver is further suggested by the peripheral type of fatty impregnation and by the observed loss of enzyme activities, in particular from the portal areas. The enzymological findings in the liver in the myopathy of 2,4-D and in muscular dystrophy of the mouse (132) cannot at present give a conclusive answer to the question, whether or not the liver would become involved in long-standing myodegenerative diseases. This applies equally to the biochemical findings in the progressive muscular dystrophy of man, which indicate a concomitant involvement of the liver (177, 178). These problems need further evaluation by clinical and experimental studies. The observation that there is an increased efflux of CPK from intact muscle fibres of the rat diaphragm on the addition of sera from patients with progressive muscular dystrophy may be mentioned in this context (285).

Relationship between the Myopathy of 2,4-D and Other Experimental Myopathies. Formal Pathogenetic Relationship to Muscular Dystrophy in Man

The present study has established the principal symptoms of the myopathy of 2,4-D as predilective involvement of white ($2B/A_m$) muscle fibres, occurrence of the earliest morphological changes in the mitochondria and the sarcoplasmic reticulum, loss of glycogen and phosphorylase activity closely related to the outcome of histological fibre damage and, finally, the sparing of the myocardium. Additional effects of this agent were found to be myotonia of skeletal muscle at early stages of intoxication (43, 268, 282), decelerated uptake of calcium by the vesicles of the sarcoplasmic reticulum (184) and, electrophysiologically, repetitive myotonic discharges (104, 268) due to the electrical hyperexcitability of the muscle fibre membrane. The pathogenetic relationship between myotonia and myopathy of 2,4-D origin is still unknown. If we compare the findings of the various experimental myopathies, it becomes evident that a close pathogenetic relationship exists between, on the one hand, the myopathy of 2,4-D and, on the other, muscular dystrophy of the mouse, myopathy of vincristine and myopathy of corticosteroids. This is particularly true of the initial proliferation of the mitochondria (49, 232, 296) and the decrease in phosphorylase activity and glycogen content of white muscle fibres in the early stages of the disease processes. The latter changes are paralleled by findings in the progressive muscular dystrophy of man (67, 115). Finally, in the experimental myopathies cited above, no involvement of the heart was observed.

The present study was concerned throughout with fully grown animals subjected to intoxication. When comparing such intoxicative myopathies with hereditary forms in animals, it must be remembered that the discontinuous and transient effect of a toxic agent cannot in principle imitate the continuous action of a genetically determined defect in the metabolism. PEARCE and WALTON (231, 232) have advanced further critical arguments against the comparison of hereditary myopathies in animals and progressive muscular dystrophy in man. Their comments are supported by some of our own histochemical findings. Thus, for instance, the ATPase pattern of the superficial layers of the gastrocnemius muscle of the rat differs from that in the corresponding parts of this muscle in man: in the animal, type $2B/A_m$ fibres prevail, as opposed to $2B/A_m$ and $2A/A_m$ fibres in the muscle of man, mitochondrial enzyme activities being low in this condition. Furthermore, marked differences in the diameter of muscle fibres of the different types can be observed in the rat, whereas in skeletal muscle of man the diameters of the various fibre types are rather more homogeneously distributed (20).

Apart from such species-dependent differences, the range of pathogenetic analogies that can be established between experimental myopathies and progressive muscular dystrophy in man is further limited by the (methodological) fact that the fibre-type composition of only a few human muscles is sufficiently well known (90, 97, 145, refs., 244, 288). Thus, in man, the question of predilective involvement of one or other fibre type cannot be answered accurately, since fibre-type composition varies considerably from superficial to deep layers within any muscle. As to the hereditary myopathies, it must be kept in mind that secondary alterations in fibres of types not primarily involved in the process will occur early in ontogenesis, thus precluding any definite statement concerning the predilective involvement of one fibre type. In addition, such functionally adaptive phenomena as a shift towards increased oxidative metabolism in the course of persistent mechanical overload of undamaged muscle fibres has to be taken into account. Experimentally, the corresponding changes towards the type of red muscle have been induced in normal muscle by means of long-lasting mechanical overload (88, 129). With these restrictions in mind, we shall attempt in the following paragraphs to apply the principal findings of our own and of other studies on experimental myopathies to the problem of progressive muscular dystrophy in man and, in particular to the Duchenne type.

In progressive muscular dystrophy of man, predilective involvement of white muscle fibres is suggested by biochemical findings, which indicate that homogenates from dystrophic muscle contain markedly lowered activities of aldolase and phosphorylase, whereas the activities of oxidative enzymes are normal or only slightly decreased (75). In further studies (145), a significant decrease was found in the activities of most glycolytic enzymes in the decantate from homogenates of muscle from patients with Duchenne muscular dystrophy. It was concluded that the oxidative metabolism would be altered by the disease process to a lesser degree than the glycolysis, thus suggesting that red and white muscle fibres could be subject to dystrophy in different ways (145). Further evidence of predilective involvement of white muscle fibres came from studies revealing lowered levels of the isozymes 4 and 5 of lactate dehydrogenase in patients as well as in preclinical cases and carriers of Duchenne dystrophy (145, refs.).

Histochemical studies dealing with questions of predilective fibre-type involvement in the muscular dystrophies of man are not numerous. DUBOWITZ and PEARSE (79) observed fibres of either type among the atrophic and hypertrophic fibres. These authors claimed that the predominant involvement of certain muscle groups in the disease, as observed clinically, would be due to variations in the numerical distribution of the fibre types in different muscles. This suggestion implies the hypothesis of predilective involvement of one fibre type in the muscular dystrophy of man. BELL and CONEN (30), in seven cases of Duchenne dystrophy, found a significant reduction (55%) in the number of type-2 (phosphorylase-positive, SDH-negative) fibres and (32%) in type-1 (phosphorylase-negative, SDH-positive) fibres as against controls, whereas the proportion of fibres related by their mitochondrial reactions to an intermediate type was increased by 71%. BALOGH and CANCILLA (20), in six biopsies of children with Duchenne muscular dystrophy, found the number of white 2A fibres decreased and that of red type-1 fibres increased. The authors suggested that this change was brought about by a transformation of 2A into type-1 fibres in the course of the disease.

An electromyographic study (72) of the mean amplitudes of the interference pattern and of the M wave following motor-nerve stimulation gave evidence of a preponderant involvement of the tibialis anterior and the gastrocnemius, which are essentially white muscles, as compared to relatively minor involvement of the red soleus muscle. Accordingly, BUCHTHAL et al. (46) recorded contractions of single muscle bundles in patients with Duchenne dystrophy and found an increase in the mean contraction times as compared to controls. Histochemically this change was correlated with an increase in the number of red C fibres. The same findings applied to neurogenic paresis (45).

With the electron microscope an increase in glycogen content and proliferation of mitochondria, followed by a reduction in number of these organelles, was observed in the early stages of muscular dystrophy (115, 211), also dilatation of the sarcoplasmic reticulum prior to myofibrillar degeneration (115, 157, 211, 229, 230, 298). Since human muscle fibre types cannot be distinguished in the electron microscope, it has not been possible to correlate strictly the electron-microscopic and the light-microscopic histochemical changes. The same kind of alteration was found in biopsies from carriers of Duchenne dystrophy (211, 255). Here focal necrosis of muscle fibres and regenerative changes could be observed (76, 120, 159, 211, 255, 304); 70% of carriers displayed increased serum CPK levels. In this group histochemical studies on muscle biopsies (77, 255) from areas outside those of focal necrosis revealed no significant alterations in the cytological structure of fibres of either type. In particular, the corresponding figures display an unaltered intermyofibrillar structure of type-2 fibres. However, these findings may not be conclusive as regards the preclinical stages of the disease, since, according to Lyon's hypothesis, the cytogenetic conditions in undamaged fibres of carriers are presumed to be rather different from those in the intact fibres of the preclinical cases. Here evidence was actually obtained of ultrastructural alterations in the intermyofibrillar space (115, 157, 211).

Besides differences in histological appearance (232), muscular dystrophy of the mouse displays electrical hyperexcitability of the muscle fibre membrane (204). This fact has been put forward as an argument against claims for similarity in muscular dystrophy of mouse and man. This argument would also apply to the hyperexcitability caused by the veratrine-like action of 2,4-D (104). However, the phenomenon of hyperexcitability of the muscle fibre membrane, giving rise in dystrophic mouse muscle to pseudomyotonic discharges with shortening of the refractory period (58), was also observed in the myopathy of vitamin-E deficiency (116) and in hereditary dystrophy in the chicken (150). Its occurrence thus is not restricted to these experimental myopathies. Pseudomyotonic discharges could also be recorded in patients with Duchenne dystrophy (44, 82,

124, 218, 251), in which shortening of both absolute and relative refractory periods of muscle contraction could be demonstrated (109). DESMEDT et al. (71) have shown that repetitive discharges and myotonic changes of contraction in the adductor pollicis muscle of Duchenne patients precede not only any clinical involvement of this muscle, but also the classic signs in the electromyogram indicative of myopathy.

In myotonic dystrophy a predilective atrophy of type-1 muscle fibres has been established (98). Hence, when seeking to establish analogies between this disease and experimental myopathies of type 2, such as the myopathy of 2,4-D, it must be remembered critically that predilective involvement of fibre types is directly contrary in both these conditions. It was claimed in the preceding chapters that the heart muscle would not be involved in myopathies of type 2. This conclusion was reached from the study of experimental myopathies in animals. The extent to which this applies to the involvement of the heart in progressive muscular dystrophy of man remains to be determined. Fairly divergent views have been proposed concerning the pathogenesis and etiology of cardiomyopathy in muscular dystrophy of man. Some workers regard cardiomyopathy as a primary symptom, that is, one immediately correlated with the disease process in skeletal muscle, while others consider that it develops as a secondary change, due to cardiopulmonary alterations arising from respiratory insufficiency, caused by the effects of the dystrophic process on the intercostal muscles and the diaphragm in advanced stages of the disease (70, 319). Cardiac involvement, supported by clinical criteria including the electrocardiogram (ECG), was reported in 25% (305) and 80% (15) of cases with muscular dystrophy. Autopsy examinations of the heart were rarely performed. In 7 patients with Duchenne dystrophy and distinct clinical signs of cardiac involvement, there was histological evidence of extensive replacement of the myocardium by connective tissue, resembling cardiac infarction (121); areas where the structure of the myocardium was preserved and with slightly enlarged nuclei could also be seen. The site of the scars was often, but not always related to blood vessels. The endocardium and epicardium were unchanged. Unlike skeletal muscle, the affected myocardium displayed no infiltration by fat cells. It must be noted that the appearance of the changes in the myocardium was different from that of the myopathic alterations of skeletal muscle that occur in the process of dystrophy. A further study (221) reported alterations in the shape and size of nuclei of the cardiac fibres in close proximity to connective tissue scars. In addition, segmental degeneration and occasional phagocytosis of muscle fibres could be observed. A marked increase in cardiac weight was found to result from lipomatosis and fibrosis of the heart muscle (153, 283). As regards the involvement of the conduction system, a single study reports granular cystic degeneration of the unstriated muscle fibres in the medial layer of the sinusoidal artery (161), the lumen of which did not appear to be occluded. Without showing a constant relationship to the vascular supply, the myofibres of the sinusoidal node were subject to disseminated degeneration. Similar alterations were observed in the fibres of the bundle of His when its interventricular course ran near septal areas of fibrosis. Vascular alterations like those observed in the sinusoidal artery could be found in the lungs, in the colon and, rarely, in skeletal muscle. The changes in the sinusoidal artery and, partly independent of these, the degeneration in the fibres of the sinusoidal node and the bundle of His were regarded as critical to the outcome of the clinically observed disturbance in the conduction system.

The occurrence of sinus tachycardia of unknown origin in patients with muscular dystrophy is well documented (121, 270, 310), this change being most outstanding in the Duchenne group (319). GILROY et al. (121), in their clinical study of 133 patients with the Duchenne type of disease, found normal ECG recordings in 32% of cases and signs of intraventricular conduction disturbances in 39%. These changes presented as a tall R wave in the right precordial leads, as incomplete right bundle-branch block (274, 284, 310), and as right cardiac hypertrophy; in 15% of the cases (121) the last two changes occurred as an isolated finding. General cardiac involvement, as indicated by ECG in 14% of cases, was constantly observed in advanced stages of the disease. The age range of normal ECG findings, with or without elevation of the R wave, was from 1 to 15 years of ongoing disease. Severe involvement of the myocardium was present at earliest after 8 years. PERLOFF et al. (235) stressed that deviations from the normal ECG pattern and changes in the QRS complex, in particular in Duchenne dystrophy, suggest cardiac involvement only if dystrophy of skeletal muscle can be clinically ascertained. In 73 patients with Duchenne muscular dystrophy, no positive correlation could be established between the kind of ECG changes seen (alterations of the QRS complex and/or complete right bundle branch block) and duration of the disease process, degree of immobilization and deformation of the thorax (274). ZELLWEGER et al. (319) found among 81 patients aged from 5 to 19 years with Duchenne muscular dystrophy unspecific ECG alterations in 85% and a tall precordial R wave, suggestive of right ventricular hypertrophy in 75%. The latter change was inconstantly combined with a deep Q wave in the left precordial leads. There appeared to be no correlation between cardiac changes and clinical criteria of the disease in skeletal muscle. The authors stressed that, although the ECG findings suggested a dystrophic cardiomyopathy, the patients presented no signs of cardiac failure.

Results of enzymological studies in blood sera of patients with Duchenne dystrophy gave no evidence of a correlation between the progression of the disorder in skeletal muscle and in the heart (178). Three out of 18 carriers with elevated CPK levels in the blood had an ECG pattern comparable to that observed in cases of frank disease (193). Some authors, although not excluding a direct involvement of the heart in the disease, have stressed that right ventricular insufficiency would result from the haemodynamic insufficiency of the pulmonary circuit caused by reduced respiratory capacities in advanced stages of the disease (70, 118, 152, 284).

Summarizing, in Duchenne muscular dystrophy considerable divergence has been reported between the type and degree of lesions of skeletal muscle and cardiac changes. Several authors (121, 178, 274, 305) have pointed out that no satisfactory qualitative and quantitative correlation can be established between the manifestations of the disease in these two types of tissue. Thus, except perhaps for the conduction system of the heart, the myocardium is not likely to be primarily involved in the dystrophic process. Indirect evidence is thus provided for the hypothesis of a predilective involvement of white fibres of skeletal muscle in muscular dystrophy of man. Studies of experimental myopathies in animals are thus of prime importance for an understanding of the pathogenesis of progressive muscular dystrophy in man.

Summary

Experimental Myopathies and Muscular Dystrophy. A Study of the
Formal Pathogenesis of Primary Myopathies as Exemplified in the
Myopathy of 2,4-Dichlorophenoxyacetic Acid

The histochemical types of muscle fibres are described and a
report presented of the histological and histochemical alterations in skeletal muscles (tibialis anterior, gastrocnemius
and soleus muscles) of rats given intraperitoneal injections
of the herbicide, 2,4-dichlorophenoxyacetic acid (2,4-D). The
liver and myocardium of the experimental animals were also
examined.

In skeletal muscle, alterations occurring acutely within 1 to
1.5 h after injection of a single dose of 300 mg/kg 2,4-D
could be distinguished from changes which developed subacutely
in the course of treatment with repeated injections of one
quarter to one half of the LD_{50} of the substance. In both conditions white (type $2B/A_m$) muscle fibres were involved predilectively. The principal histochemical effect of acute intoxication observed was leakage of phosphorylase and glycogen from
white muscle fibres, whereas some of the red fibres (type $2A/C_m$)
showed an increase in primary glycogen and phosphorylase activity. These changes, which must be considered nonspecific, were
established by use of a gelatin incubation technique. They
occurred as typical findings in the middle and deep areas of
the anterior tibial muscle. In other muscles or different
layers of the same muscle, these changes varied considerably
in degree. Thus the gastrocnemius and soleus muscles displayed
only minor or no alterations. These differences could represent
a different time course in the intoxication of the respective
muscles. The histological structure and histochemical activities of diaphorases and of α-glycerophosphate dehydrogenase
were unaffected.

Under conditions of subacute intoxication, a myopathy of white
type-$2B/A_m$ fibres developed. Contrary to the findings in the
acute experiment, the earliest changes were seen, not in phosphorylase, but in mitochondria and the sarcoplasmic reticulum
of white fibres. As shown by histochemical dehydrogenase reactions, these consisted of disorganization of the perimyofibrillar network, suggestive of mitochondrial swelling. Segmental
swelling of type-2 fibres was the first histological sign of
fibre damage; it was always accompanied by loss of glycogen
and of phosphorylase, glycogensynthetase and succinodehydrogenase activities. These changes preceded fibre necrosis.

At the height of the disease process, extensive myopathic changes
could be observed in addition to a few alterations suggesting
neurogenic atrophy of single muscle fibres. Atrophy was considered to be consequent to denervation, caused at early stages
of the disease by myopathic alterations near the axon terminals
of the respective muscle fibres; in these, myopathic changes
were not outstanding.

In the soleus muscle necrosis could be observed only at the
height of the disease process in single red ($2A/C_m$) fibres,
whereas the bulk of intermediate type-1/B_m fibres of this muscle
did not show any alterations.

When treatment was halted, a complete reversal of the alterations occurred within 10 to 14 days, with myopathic changes
receding faster than atrophic ones. Besides the qualitative
restitution of the structure of type-2 fibres, quantitative
regeneration phenomena, i.e. longitudinal division of muscle
fibres, could be observed.

Corresponding studies of liver specimens revealed loss of
glycogen and of phosphorylase activity from portal areas in
the early stages of the disease, and in the later stages an
additional decrease in dehydrogenase activities, together
with intracellular deposition of fat droplets in the periphery
of the liver lobules.

The myocardium of the ventricles, which is histochemically a
red (type-$2C/C_m$) muscle, did not show any clear alterations.
In particular, no histological lesions could be detected. The
conduction system of the heart was not examined.

The cytological alterations of white muscle fibres early in
the disease are regarded as resulting from compensatory activation of the oxidative metabolism, due to drug-induced inhibition of glycolysis in these fibres. The succeeding histological changes, i.e. swelling and necrosis of white ($2B/A_m$)
muscle fibres, are accompanied histochemically by a loss of
glycolytic and oxidative capacities. Thus, these changes indicate the point at which aerobic mechanisms can no longer
compensate for the defect of glycolysis. The experimentally
established vulnerability of white muscle fibres could be
explained on this basis.

The account of the findings in the experiments with 2,4-D is
preceded by a survey of the literature on experimental myopathies. Special attention is given to reports of predilective
involvement of one fibre type or of heart muscle. Myopathies
of type 2 (to which that of 2,4-D belongs) without involvement of the myocardium can be distinguished from myopathies
of type 1 (to which that of chloroquine belongs) in which
the heart muscle is involved.

As regards the formal pathogenesis, the myopathy of 2,4-D in
the rat is related to the myopathy of vincristine in this
species and to hereditary myopathy in the mouse.

The concepts derived from the studies in experimental myopathies
are extended to problems of Duchenne muscular dystrophy in man.
Arguments are put forward suggesting that in this disease white
(type-2) fibres are also predilectively involved. Indirect evidence that this is so can be obtained from findings indicating
that the myocardium is not altered until late in the disease.

On the whole, the myopathy of 2,4-D can be regarded as a suitable
model for studying primary myopathies in animals and man.

In addition, histochemical findings are presented on the in-vitro
effects of 2,4-D on muscle phosphorylase. A gelatin incubation
technique was used to show that the histochemical activity of
phosphorylase declines as an effect of 2,4-D administration.
Evidence is presented indicating that this is not due to direct
action of 2,4-D on the enzyme but to inhibition at some point
of the phosphorylase activating system.

Zusammenfassung

In der vorliegenden Arbeit wird nach einer Darstellung der histochemischen Typologie der Muskelfasern über die histologischen
und histochemischen Veränderungen berichtet, die im Skelettmuskel (M. tibialis ant. und M. triceps surae) der Ratte nach intra-
peritonealer Gabe von 2,4-Dichlorphenoxyacetat (2,4-D) auftreten.
Paralleluntersuchungen wurden an Leber und Kammermyokard der Ver-
suchstiere durchgeführt.

Es wird unterschieden zwischen den akuten Veränderungen im Skelettmuskel, wie sie 1 - 1,5 Std nach einmaliger Injektion von 300 mg/kg
2,4-D auftreten sowie subakut einsetzenden Veränderungen, die nach
wiederholter Injektion von 1/4 - 1/2 LD_{50} der Substanz beobachtet
werden. In beiden Fällen werden die "weißen" (Typ $2B/A_m$) Fasern
prädilektiv geschädigt.

Bei akuter Intoxikation wurde im Stadium der Myotonie histochemisch
mittels Geltechnik ein Abstrom von Phosphorylase und Glykogen aus
weißen ($2B/A_m$) Muskelfasern nachgewiesen; in einem Teil der roten
(Typ $2A/C_m$) Fasern hingegen kam es zu einer Zunahme der Phosphorylase-Aktivität und des Glykogengehaltes. Diese, nicht spezifischen
Veränderungen sind sowohl in verschiedenen Tiefen eines Muskels
als auch in verschiedenen Muskeln unterschiedlich ausgeprägt.
Der typische Befund wurde in der mittleren und tiefen Schicht
des M. tibialis ant. erhoben, während der M. gastrocnemius nur
schwache und inkonstante Veränderungen zeigte. Als Ursache dieses
differenten Verhaltens ist möglicherweise ein unterschiedlicher
zeitlicher Verlauf der Schädigung in den einzelnen Muskeln anzu-
sehen. - Die Veränderungen sind innerhalb von höchstens 24 Std
voll reversibel. Histologische Faserstruktur sowie histochemische
Aktivitäten der Diaphorasen und der menadionabhängigen α-Glycero-
phosphat-Dehydrogenase bleiben unverändert.

Bei der subakuten Intoxikation mit 2,4-D entwickelt sich eine
Myopathie vom Typ 2, wobei erste Veränderungen selektiv eben-
falls in den weißen ($2B/A_m$) Fasern auftreten. Hierbei handelt
es sich histochemisch jedoch primär nicht um Aktivitätsänderun-
gen der Phosphorylase, sondern um Zeichen einer Proliferation
von Mitochondrien und um Veränderungen am sarkoplasmatischen
Retikulum dieses Fasertyps.

Die primären Veränderungen in weißen ($2B/A_m$) Fasern bestehen
in einer Desorganisation der perimyofibrillären Struktur und
lassen sich lichtmikroskopisch mittels der histochemischen De-
hydrogenasenachweises darstellen. Als erste histologisch faß-
bare Veränderung tritt segmentäre Schwellung von $2B/A_m$-Fasern
ein, mit Verlust von Glykogen, von Phosphorylase-, Glykogen-

synthetase- und Succinodehydrogenase-Aktivitäten sowie an-
schließender Fasernekrose. Im Vollstadium der Erkrankung fin-
den sich neben myopathisch veränderten spärliche atrophische
Muskelfasern, deren Entwicklung als Folge einer Schädigung
ihres terminalen Axons durch myopathische Veränderungen in
der Nachbarschaft gedeutet wird. Diese treten in den atropischen
Muskelfasern zurück. - Innerhalb von 10-14 Tagen nach Absetzen
der Behandlung kommt es zu einer vollen Remission der Veränderungen. Hierbei regenerieren myopatisch veränderte Fasern rascher
als atropische. Neben der qualitativen Regeneration der einzelnen Muskelfaser werden Zeichen einer numerischen Regeneration
durch Längsspaltung beobachtet. Im (roten) M. soleus lassen
sich lediglich im Vollstadium der Erkrankung vereinzelte Ne-
krosen der hier spärlich vertretenen $2A/C_m$-Fasern nachweisen,
während der Hauptfasertyp $1/C_m$ völlig verschont bleibt.

Paralleluntersuchungen an der Leber erwiesen einen vorwiegend
portalen Glykogenverlust mit paralleler Abnahme der Phosphorylase-Aktivität im Frühstadium, im Vollstadium zusätzlich eine
Abnahme der Dehydrogenase-Aktivitäten im portalen Bereich und
eine feintropfige Verfettung der Läppchenperipherie.

Das Myokard der Herzkammern, histochemisch ein roter Muskel
vom Typ $2C/C_m$, zeigte auch in schweren Erkrankungsstadien
keine eindeutigen Veränderungen, insbesondere keine histologischen Schäden. Das Reizleitungssystem wurde nicht unter-
sucht.

Die zytologischen Frühveränderungen in den weißen ($2B/A_m$)
Fasern des Skelettmuskels werden gedeutet als Ausdruck einer
kompensativen Aktivierung des oxidativen Stoffwechsels bei
partieller Schädigung der Glykolyse dieser Fasern. Das Auftreten histologisch faßbarer Schäden (Faserschwellung) in
weißen ($2B/A_m$) Muskelfasern geht histochemisch mit einem Verlust anaerober und aerober Stoffwechselkapazitäten der Zelle
einher. Es kennzeichnet den Zeitpunkt, an welchem die kompensativen (aeroben) Stoffwechselmechanismen der weißen Muskelfaser versagen. Aus diesem Verhalten erhellt die höhere Vul-
nerabilität der weißen, vorwiegend anaeroben, gegenüber den
roten aeroben (oder gemischt anaerob-aeroben) Muskelfasern
auch bei dieser experimentellen Myopathie.

Dem Bericht über die eigenen Untersuchungen ist eine Literatur-
übersicht über die bisher bekannten experimentellen Myopathieformen vorangestellt, wobei die Gesichtspunkte der prädilekti-
ven Schädigung eines Fasertyps sowie der Herzbeteiligung be-
sonders berücksichtigt werden. Im Ergebnis lassen sich den
Myopathien vom Typ 2 (z.B. 2,4-D-Myopathie) ohne Beteiligung
des Herzmuskels Myopathien vom Typ 1 (z.B. Chlorochin-Myopathie)
mit primärer Herzbeteiligung gegenüberstellen. Formalpathogene-
tisch ist die 2,4-D-Myopathie u.a. der Vincristin-Myopathie der
Ratte sowie der erheblichen Dystrophie der Maus eng verwandt.

Die an den tierexperimentellen Myopathieformen gewonnenen Vor-
stellungen werden mit Befunden bei Duchennescher Muskeldystrophie des Menschen verglichen. Auch hierbei sprechen zahlreiche
Argumente für eine prädilektive Schädigung weißer (Typ $2/A_m$)

Muskelfasern. Ferner findet sich auch bei dieser Erkrankungs-
form erst in relativ späten Verlaufsstadien eine Beteiligung
des Myokards am dystrophischen Prozeß.

Insgesamt erweist sich die 2,4-D-Myopathie als ein geeignetes
tierexperimentelles Modell zum Studium der formalen Pathogenese
primärer Myopathien von Mensch und Tier.

Im weiteren Rahmen des Themas werden neue histochemische Befunde zur in-vitro-Wirkung von 2,4-D auf die Phosphorylase-Aktivität des Skelettmuskels vorgelegt. Nach diesen, mit kriti-
scher histochemischer Technik erzielten Ergebnissen bewirkt
2,4-D in vitro eine Erniedrigung der Phosphorylase-Aktivität,
wobei der Angriffsort der Substanz nicht an der Phosphorylase
selbst, sondern am Phosphorylase-aktivierenden System zu suchen
ist.

I would like to thank J.T. SWANN for his careful revision of
the English text.

References

1. ADAMS, R.D., DENNY-BROWN, D., PEARSON, C.M.: Diseases of muscle. 2nd ed.. New York: Harper & Row 1962.
2. AFIFI, A.K., BERGMAN, R.A., HARVEY, C.J.: Steroid myopathy. Clinic, histologic and cytologic observations. Johns Hopkins Med. J. $\underline{123}$, 158-174 (1968).
3. AFIFI, A.K., BERGMAN, R.A.: Steroid myopathy. A study of the evolution of the muscle lesion in rabbits. Johns Hopkins Med. J. $\underline{124}$, 66-68 (1969).
4. AGUAYO, A.J., HUDGSON, P.: Observations on the short-term effects of chloroquine on skeletal muscle. An experimental study in the rabbit. J. Neurol. Sci. $\underline{11}$, 301-326 (1970).
5. ALBUQUERQUE, E.X., WARNICK, J.E.: Electrophysiological observations in normal and dystrophic chicken muscles. Science $\underline{172}$, 1260-1262 (1971).
6. ALOISI, M., ASCENZI, A., BONETTI, C.: Submicroscopical changes in muscles of vitamin-E-deficient rabbits. J. Path. Bact. $\underline{64}$, 321-327 (1952).
7. ALOISI, M., MARGRETH, A.: The question of glycolytic enzymes localization in the skeletal muscle fiber and its bearing upon certain aspects of muscle disease. In: Exploratory concepts in muscular dystrophy and related disorders (ed. A.T. MILHORAT), p. 305-317. Excerpta Med. Found. Intern. Congr. Ser. No. 147, Amsterdam, New York, London, Paris, Milan, Tokyo, Buenos Aires 1967.
8. ANGELINI, C., DIMAURO, S., MARGRETH, A.: Relationship of serum enzyme changes to muscle damage in vitamin-E-deficiency of the rabbit. Sperimentale $\underline{118}$, 349-370 (1969).
9. ASHMORE, C.E., SOMES, R.G., Jr., VASINGTON, F.D.: Relative distributions of myoglobin derivatives in breast muscle of chickens with hereditary muscular dystrophy. Proc. Soc. exp. Biol. Med. $\underline{122}$, 1104-1107 (1966).
10. ASHMORE, C.E., SOMES, R.G., Jr.: Delay of hereditary muscular dystrophy of the chicken by oxygen therapy: histology. Proc. Soc. exp. Biol. Med. $\underline{128}$, 103-107 (1968).
11. ASHMORE, C.E., DOERR, L.: Phosphorylase in skeletal muscle of normal and selected lines of dystrophic chickens. Proc. Soc. exp. Biol. Med. $\underline{137}$, 1066-1068 (1971).
12. ASHMORE, C.E., DOERR, L.: Postnatal development of fiber types in normal dystrophic skeletal muscle of the chick. Exp. Neurol. $\underline{30}$, 431-446 (1971).
13. ASMUNDSON, V.S., JULIAN, L.M.: Inherited muscle abnormality in the domestic fowl. J. Hered. $\underline{47}$, 248-252 (1956).
14. ASMUNDSON, V.S., KRATZER, F.H., JULIAN, L.M.: Inherited myopathy in the chicken. Ann. N.Y. Acad. Sci. $\underline{138}$, 49-58 (1966).

15. BAGHIRZADE, M.F., WEISS, V.: Myokardbeteiligung bei progressiver Muskeldystrophie. Dtsch. Med. Wschr. 95, 1447-1450 (1970).
16. BAJUSZ, E., HOMBURGER, F., BAKER, J.R., OPIE, L.H.: The heart muscle in muscular dystrophy with special reference to involvement of the cardiovascular system in the hereditary myopathy of the hamster. Ann. N.Y. Acad. Sci. 138, 223-229 (1966).
17. BAJUSZ, E., BAKER, J.R., NIXON, C.W., HOMBURGER, F.: Spontaneous hereditary myocardial degeneration and congestive heart failure in a strain of syrian hamsters. Ann. N.Y. Acad. Sci. 156, 105-129 (1969).
18. BAKER, N.: Supersensitivity to anticholinesterases of isolated nerve-muscle preparation from hereditarily dystrophic mice. J. Pharmacol. exp. Ther. 141, 223-229 (1963).
19. BALOGH, K., Jr., PRAGAY, D.A., HOYT, R.F., Jr.: Myocardial enzymes in plasmocid-poisoned rabbits. A correlative histochemical and biochemical study. Lab. Invest. 16, 211-219 (1967).
20. BALOGH, .R., CANCILLA, P.A.: An appraisal of histochemical fiber types in Duchenne muscular dystrophy. Neurology (Minneap.) 22, 1243-1252 (1972).
21. BANKER, B.Q.: A phase and electron microscopic study of dystrophic muscle. I. The pathological changes in the two-week-old Bar Harbor 129 dystrophic mouse. J. Neuropath. exp. Neurol. 26, 259-275 (1967).
22. BANKER, B.Q.: A phase and electron microscopic study of dystrophic muscle. II. The pathological changes in the newborn Bar Harbor 129 dystrophic mouse. J. Neuropath. exp. Neurol. 27, 183-209 (1968).
23. BANKER, B.Q., DENNY-BROWN, D.: A study of denervated muscle in normal and dystrophic mice. J. Neuropath. exp. Neurol. 18, 517-530 (1959).
24. BÁRÁNY, M.: Adenosine triphosphatase activity of myosin correlated with speed of muscle shortening. J. gen. Physiol. 50, 197-218 (1967).
25. BÁRÁNY, M., CLOSE, R.I.: The transformation of myosin in cross-innervated rat muscles. J. Physiol. (Lond.) 213, 455-474 (1971).
26. BARNARD, R.J., EDGERTON, V.R., FURUKAWA, T., PETER, J.B.: Histochemical, biochemical and contractile properties of red, white and intermediate fibers. Amer. J. Physiol. 220, 410-414 (1971).
27. BASS, A., BRDICZKA, D., EYER, P., HOFER, S., PETTE, D.: Metabolic differentiation of distinct muscle types at the level of enzymatic organization. Europ. J. Biochem. 10, 198-206 (1969).
28. BEATTY, C.H., BASINGER, G.M., BOCEK, R.M.: Pentose cycle activity in muscle from fetal, neonatal and infant rhesus monkeys. Arch. Biochem. Biophys. 117, 275-281 (1966).
29. BECKMANN, R., BILLICH, C.: Die Leber bei der Dystrophia musculorum progressiva (Erb). (Biochemische und morphologische Befunde). Med. Welt (Stuttg.) 19, 1085-1094 (1962).
30. BELL, C.D., CONEN, P.E.: Histochemical fibre "types" in Duchenne muscular dystrophy. J. neurol. Sci. 10, 163-172 (1970).

31. BLANCHAER, M.C., WIJHE, M., van, MOZERSKY, D.: The oxidation of lactate and α-glycerophosphate by red and white skeletal muscle: I. Quantitative studies. J. Histochem. Cytochem. <u>11</u>, 500-504 (1963).

32. BOWDEN, D.H., GOYER, R.A.: Drug-induced muscle necrosis with massive taurinuria. Arch. Path. <u>74</u>, 137-141 (1962).

33. BRADLEY, W.G.: The neuromyopathy of vincristine in the guinea pig. An electrophysiological and pathological study. J. neurol. Sci. <u>10</u>, 133-162 (1970).

34. BRAY, G.M., BANKER, B.Q.: An ultrastructural study of degeneration and necrosis of muscle in the dystrophic mouse. Acta Neuropath. (Berlin) <u>15</u>, 34-44 (1970).

35. BRODY, I.A., ENGEL, W.K.: Effects of phenazine methosulfate in histochemistry. J. Histochem. Cytochem. <u>12</u>, 628-629 (1964).

36. BROOKE, M.H., ENGEL, W.K.: Use of phenazine methosulfate in enzyme histochemistry of human muscle biopsies. Neurology <u>16</u>, 986-993 (1966).

37. BROOKE, M.H., KAISER, K.K.: Some comments on the histochemical characterization of muscle adenosine triphosphatase. J. Histochem. Cytochem. <u>17</u>, 431-432 (1969).

38. BROOKE, M.H., KAISER, K.K.: Muscle fiber types. How many and what kind. Arch. Neurol. <u>23</u>, 369-379 (1970).

39. BRUST, M.: Contraction enhancement in skeletal muscles of normal and dystrophic mice. Amer. J. Physiol. <u>208</u>, 425-430 (1965).

40. BRUST, M.: Combined effects of nitrate and caffeine on contractions of skeletal muscles. Amer. J. Physiol. <u>208</u>, 431-435 (1965).

41. BRUST, M.: Relative resistance to dystrophy of slow skeletal muscle of the mouse. Amer. J. Physiol. <u>210</u>, 445-451 (1966).

42. BRUST, M.: Agents which affect excitation-contraction coupling in normal and dystrophic muscle. Fed. Proc. <u>28</u>, 1649-1656 (1969).

43. BUCHER, N.L.R.: Effects of 2,4-dichlorophenoxyacetic acid on experimental animals. Proc. Soc. exp. Biol. (N.Y.) <u>63</u>, 204-205 (1946).

44. BUCHTHAL, F., ROSENFALCK, P.: Electrophysiological aspects of myopathy with particular reference to progressive muscular dystrophy. In: Muscular dystrophy in man and animals (ed. G.H. BOURNE, M.N. GOLARZ). Basel, New York: Karger 1963.

45. BUCHTHAL, F., SCHMALBRUCH, H., KAMIENIECKA, Z.: Contraction times and fiber types in neurogenic paresis. Neurology (Minneap.) <u>21</u>, 58-67 (1971).

46. BUCHTHAL, F., SCHMALBRUCH, H., KAMIENIECKA, Z.: Contraction times and fiber types in patients with progressive muscular dystrophy. Neurology (Minneap.) <u>21</u>, 131-139 (1971).

47. BÜCHNER, F.: Qualitative morphology of heart failure. In: Meth. Achievm. exp. Path., Vol. 5 (ed. E. BAJUSZ, G. JASMIN), pp. 60-120. Basel, New York: Karger 1971.

48. BULLER, A.J., MOMMAERTS, W.F.H.M., SERAYDARIAN, K.: Enzymic properties of myosin in fast and slow twitch muscles of the cat following cross-innervation. J. Physiol. (Lond.) <u>205</u>, 581-597 (1969).

49. BULLOCK, G.R., CHRISTIAN, R.A., PETERS, R.F., WHITE, A.M.: Rapid mitochondrial enlargement in muscle as a response to triamcinolone acetonide and its relationship to the ribosomal defect. Biochem. Pharmacol. $\underline{20}$, 943-954 (1971).

50. BUNYAN, J., GREEN, J., DIPLOCK, A.T.: Lysosomal enzymes and vitamin-E deficiency. 3. Liver necrosis and testicular degeneration in the rat. Brit. J. Nutr. $\underline{21}$, 147-154 (1967).

51. BURKE, R.E., LEVINE, D.N., ZAJAC, F.E., TSAIRIS, P., ENGEL, W.K.: Mammalian motor units: physiological-histochemical correlation in three types in cat gastrocnemius. Science $\underline{174}$, 709-712 (1971).

52. CANAL, N., FRATTOLA, L.: Studies on the pentose phosphate pathway in hereditary muscular dystrophy in mice. Med. Exp. $\underline{7}$, 27-31 (1962).

53. CANAL, N., FRATTOLA, L., POLONI, A.E.: Studies on the "Pentose phosphate pathway" in denervated skeletal muscle. Med. Exp. $\underline{10}$, 79-84 (1964).

54. CARDINET, G.H., TYLER, S., JULIAN, L.M.: Ultrastructural observations of vacuoles in hereditary avian muscular dystrophy. Anat. Rec. $\underline{157}$, 224 (1967).

55. CHOR, H., DOLKART, R.E.: Experimental muscular dystrophy in the guinea pig. A nutritional myo-degeneration. Arch. Pathol. $\underline{27}$, 497-509 (1939).

56. CLARKE, J.T.R., KARPATI, G., CARPENTER, S., WOLFE, L.S.: The effect of vincristine on skeletal muscle in the rat. A correlative histochemical, ultrastructural and chemical study. J. Neuropath. exp. Neurol. $\underline{31}$, 247-266 (1972).

57. COLEMAN, D.L., ASHWORTH, M.E.: Incorporation of glycine-1-C^{14} into nucleic acids and proteins of mice with hereditary muscular dystrophy. Amer. J. Physiol. $\underline{197}$, 839-841 (1959).

58. CONRAD, J.T., GLASER, G.H.: Bioelectric properties of dystrophic mammalian muscle. Arch. Neurol. (Chicago) $\underline{5}$, 46-57 (1961).

59. CONRAD, J.T., GLASER, G.H.: Neuromuscular fatigue in dystrophic muscle. Nature $\underline{196}$, 997-998 (1962).

60. CONRAD, J.T., GLASER, G.H.: Spontaneous activity at myoneural junction in dystrophic muscle. Arch. Neurol. (Chicago) $\underline{11}$, 310-316 (1964).

61. COOPER, C.C., CASSENS, R.G., BRISKEY, E.J.: Capillary distribution and fiber characteristics in skeletal muscle of stress-susceptible animals. J. Food Sci. $\underline{34}$, 299-302 (1969).

62. COSMOS, E.: A study of phosphorylase activity in muscle of normal and dystrophic chickens. J. Histochem. Cytochem. $\underline{13}$, 704-705 (1965).

63. COSMOS, E.: Enzymatic activity of differentiating muscle fibers. I. Development of phosphorylase in muscles of the domestic fowl. Developmental Biol. $\underline{13}$, 163-181 (1966).

64. COSMOS, E., BUTLER, J.: Differentiation of fiber types in muscle of normal and dystrophic chickens. A quantitative and histochemical study of the ontogeny of muscle enzymes. In: Exploratory concepts in muscular dystrophy and related disorders (ed. A.T. MILHORAT). Amsterdam: Excerpta Medica Intern. Congr. Ser. No. 147, 1967.

65. COSMOS, E., BUTLER, F., SCOTT, R.: Phosphorylase activity in differentiating muscle fibers of the domestic fowl. J. Histochem. Cytochem. 13, 719-720 (1965)(Proceedings).

66. D'AGOSTINO, A.N.: An electron microscopic study of skeletal and cardiac muscle of the rat poisoned by plasmocid. Lab. Invest. 12, 1060-1071 (1963).

67. D'AGOSTINO, A.N., CHIGA, M.: Cortisone myopathy in rabbits; a light and electron microscopic study. Neurology (Minneap.) 16, 257-263 (1966).

68. D'AGOSTINO, A.N., CHIGA, M.: Morphologic changes in cardiac and skeletal muscle induced by corticosteroids. Ann. N.Y. Acad. Sci. 138, 73-81 (1966).

69. DALGAARD-MIKKELSEN, S., POULSEN, E.: Toxicology of herbicides. Pharmacol. Rev. 14, 225-250 (1962).

70. DEMANY, M.A., ZIMMERMANN, H.A.: Progressive muscular dystrophy. Hemodynamic, angiographic, and pathological study of a patient with myocardial involvement. Circulation 40, 377-384 (1969).

71. DESMEDT, J.E., EMERYK, B., will coll., RENOIRTE, P., HAINAUT, K.: Disorders of muscle contraction processes in sex-linked (Duchenne) muscular dystrophy, with correlative electromyographic study of myopathic involvement in small hand muscles. Amer. J. Med. 45, 853-872 (1968).

72. DIMITRIJEVIĆ, M.R., GRAČANIN, F.: Differential involvement of tibialis anterior, gastrocnemius and soleus in muscular dystrophy. J. Neurol. Sci. 6, 105-115 (1968).

73. DREYFUS, J.C.: Problems in the biochemistry of progressive muscular dystrophy. In: Research in muscular dystrophy (Proc. 2nd sympos. Jan. 1963). London: Pitman Medical 1963.

74. DREYFUS, J.C., SCHAPIRA, G., SCHAPIRA, F.: Biochemical study of muscle in progressive muscular dystrophy. J. Clin. Invest. 33, 794-797 (1954).

75. DREYFUS, J.C., SCHAPIRA, G.: Biochemistry of hereditary myopathies. Springfield, Ill.: Charles C. Thomas 1962.

76. DUBOWITZ, V.: Myopathic changes in muscular dystrophy carriers. Proc. Roy. Soc. J. Med. 56, 810-812 (1963).

77. DUBOWITZ, V.: Developing and diseased muscle. A histochemical study. London: Heimann 1968.

78. DUBOWITZ, V., PEARSE, A.G.E.: A comparative histochemical study of oxidative enzyme and phosphorylase activity in skeletal muscle. Histochemie 2, 105-117 (1960).

79. DUBOWITZ, V., PEARSE, A.G.E.: Enzymic activity of normal and dystrophic human muscle. A histochemical study. J. Path. Bact. 81, 365-378 (1961).

80. DURACK, D.T., GUBBAY, S.S., KAKULAS, B.A.: Electrophysiological studies in the rottnest quokka with nutritional myopathy. Aust. J. exp. Biol. Med. Sci. 47, 581-588 (1969).

81. EADIE, M.J., FERRIER, T.M.: Chloroquine myopathy. J. Neurol. Neurosurg. Psychiat. 29, 331-337 (1966).

82. EATON, L.M., LAMBERT, E.H.: Electromyography and electric stimulation of nerves in diseases of motor units; observations on myasthenic syndrome associated with malignant tumors. J.A.M.A. 163, 1117-1124 (1957).

83. EBERSTEIN, A., GOODGOLD, J.: Induced myotonia in fast and slow muscles of the rat. Experientia (Basel) 25, 1269-1270 (1969).

84. ECKNER, F.A.C., RIEBE, B.H., MOULDER, P.V., BLACKSTONE, E.H.: Polysaccharide synthesis in tissue sections. Evaluation of methods as an example of quality control in histochemistry. Histochemie 19, 340-354 (1969).
85. EDGERTON, V.R., SIMPSON, D.R.: The intermediate muscle fiber of rats and guinea pigs. J. Histochem. Cytochem. 17, 828-838 (1969).
86. EDGERTON, V.R., GERCHMAN, L., CARROW, R.: Histochemical changes in rat skeletal muscle after exercise. Exp. Neurol. 24, 110-123 (1969).
87. EDGERTON, V.R., BARNARD, R.J., PETER, J.B., SIMPSON, D.R., GILLEPSIE, C.A.: Response of muscle glycogen and phosphorylase to electrical stimulation in trained and non-trained guinea pigs. Exp. Neurol. 27, 46-56 (1970).
88. EDGERTON, V.R., BARNARD, R.J.: Dynamic and metabolic relationship in the rat extensor digitorum longus muscle. Exp. Neurol. 30, 374-376 (1971).
89. EDSTRÖM, L., KUGELBERG, E.: Histochemical composition, distribution of fibres and fatigability of single motor units. Anterior tibial muscle of the rat. J. Neurol. Neurosurg. Psychiat. 31, 424-433 (1968).
90. EDSTRÖM, L., NYSTRÖM, B.: Histochemical types and sizes of fibers in normal human muscle. Acta Neurol. Scand. 45, 257-269 (1969).
91. EINARSON, L., RINGSTED, A.: Effect of chronic vitamin-E deficiency on the nervous system and the skeletal musculature of adult rats. Copenhagen: Levin and Munksgaard 1939.
92. ELLIS, J.T.: Studies on the nature and pathogenesis of muscular degeneration in cortisone-treated rabbits. Bull. N.Y. Acad. Med. 29, 814-817 (1953).
93. ELLIS, J.T.: Necrosis and regeneration of skeletal muscles in cortisone-treated rabbits. Amer. J. Path. 32, 993-1013 (1956).
94. ENGEL, W.K.: The essentiality of histo- and cytochemical studies of skeletal muscle in the investigation of neuromuscular disease. Neurology (Minneap.) 12, 778-794 (1962).
95. ENGEL, W.K.: Diseases of the neuromuscular junction and muscle. In: Neurohistochemistry. Amsterdam: Elsevier 1965.
96. ENGEL, W.K.: The multiplicity of pathologic reactions of human skeletal muscle. Proc. 5th Internat. Congr. Neuropathol. Zürich, p. 613-624. Amsterdam: Excerpta Medica 1965.
97. ENGEL, W.K.: Selective and nonselective susceptibility of muscle fiber types. Arch.Neurol (Chicago) 22, 97-117 (1970).
98. ENGEL, W.K., BROOKE, M.H.: Histochemistry of myotonic disorders. In: Progressive Muskeldystrophie, Myotonie, Myastenie (ed. E. KUHN), pp. 203-222. Berlin, Heidelberg, New York: Springer 1966.
99. ENGEL, W.K., BROOKE, M.H.: Muscle biopsy as a clinical diagnostic aid. In: Neurological Diagnostic Techniques (ed. W.S. FIELDS). Springfield, Ill.: Ch.C. Thomas 1966.
100. ENGEL, W.K., CUNNINGHAM, G.G.: Rapid examination of muscle tissue. An improved trichrome method for fresh-frozen biopsy sections. Neurology (Minneap.) 13, 919-923 (1963).

101. ERBSLÖH, F.: Histo- und biochemische Befunde bei dystrophischen Myopathien. Dtsch. Z. Nervenheilk. 173, 503-516 (1955).
102. EVANS, H.M., EMERSON, G.A., TELFORD, I.R.: Degeneration of cross-striated musculature in vitamin-E-low rats. Proc. Soc. exp. Biol. Med. 38, 625-627 (1938).
103. EWEN, L.M., JENKINS, K.J.: Antidystrophic effect of selenium and other agents on chicks from vitamin-E depleted hens. J. Nutr. 93, 470-474 (1967).
104. EYZAGUIRRE, L., FOLK, B.P., ZIERLER, K.L., LILIENTHAL, J.L.: Experimental myotonia and repetitive phenomena: The veratrinic effects of 2,4-dichlorophenoxyacetate (2,4-D) in the rat. Amer. J. Physiol. 155, 69-77 (1948).
105. FAHIMI, H.D., AMARASINGHAM, C.R.: Cytochemical localization of lactic dehydrogenase in white skeletal muscle. J. Cell Biol. 22, 29-48 (1964).
106. FAHIMI, H.D., KARNOVSKY, M.J.: Cytochemical localization of two glycolytic dehydrogenases in white skeletal muscle. J. Cell Biol. 29, 113-128 (1966).
107. FAHIMI, H.D., ROY, P.: Cytochemical localization of lactate dehydrogenase in muscular dystrophy of the mouse. Science 152, 1761-1763 (1966).
108. FARLEY, T.M., SCHOLLER, J., FOLKERS, K.: Research on coenzyme Q and muscular dystrophy. In: Exploratory Concepts in Muscular Dystrophy and Related Disorders (ed. A.T. MILHORAT), pp. 378-386. Amsterdam: Excerpta Medica 1967.
109. FARMER, T.W., BUCHTHAL, F., ROSENFALCK, P.: Refractory and irresponsive periods of muscle in progressive muscular dystrophy and paresis due to lower motor neuron involvement. Neurology 9, 747-756 (1959).
110. FASOLD, H.: Pers. comm. (1967).
111. FENNELL, R.A., WEST, W.T.: Oxidative and hydrolytic enzymes of homozygous dystrophic and heterozygous muscle of the house mouse. J. Histochem. Cytochem. 11, 374-382 (1963).
112. FISCHER, R., BENITEZ, L.: Der histochemische Nachweis der Laktatdehydrogenase in roten und weißen Muskelfasern verschiedener Laboratoriumstiere. Naturwissenschaften 24, 638-639 (1964).
113. FOLKERS, K.: Survey on the vitamin aspects of coenzyme Q. Intern. Z. Vitaminforsch. 39, 334-352 (1969).
114. FORBES, M.S., SPERELAKIS, N.: Cardiomyopathy in the dystrophic mouse. In: Cardiomyopathies (ed. E. BAJUSZ, G. RONA), pp. 455-465. Baltimore: University Park Press 1973.
115. FREUND-MÖLBERT, E.: Feinstrukturelle Veränderungen bei der Muskeldystrophie. In: H. HEYCK, G. LAUDAHN: Die progressive-dystrophischen Myopathien, p. 119-138. Berlin, Heidelberg, New York: Springer 1969.
116. FUDEMA, J.J., OESTER, Y.T., FIZZELL, J.A., GATZ, A.J.: Electrical activity of striated muscle in experimental vitamin-E deficiency. Amer. J. Physiol. 198, 123-127 (1960).
117. FUJISAWA, K., SHIRAKI, H., KATSUI, G.: Early phase of axonal dystrophy in vitamin-E deficient rats. Proc. VIth Intern. Congr. Neuropathol. Paris, 1970.

118. GAILANI, S., DONOWSKI, T., FISHER, D.: Muscular dystrophy. Catheterization studies indicating latent congestive heart failure. Circulation 17, 581-588 (1958).
119. GARCIA-BUÑUEL, L., GARCIA-BUÑUEL, V.M.: Connective tissue and the pentose phosphate pathway in normal and denervated muscle. Nature 213, 913-914 (1967).
120. GARDNER-MEDWIN, D.: Studies of the carrier state in the Duchenne type of muscular dystrophy. 2. Quantitative electromyography as a method of carrier detection. J. Neurol. Neurosurg. Psychiat. 31, 124-134 (1968).
121. GILROY, J., CAHALAN, J.L., BERGMAN, R., NEWMAN, M.: Cardiac and pulmonary complications in Duchenne's progressive muscular dystrophy. Circulation 27, 484-493 (1963).
122. GIRKIN, G., FITCH, C.D., DINNING, J.S.: Nucleic acid metabolism in mice with hereditary muscular dystrophy. Arch. Biochem. 98, 224-228 (1962).
123. GLASER, G.H., SEASHORE, M.R.: End-plate cholinesterase in dystrophic muscle. Nature 214, 1351 (1967).
124. GOODGOLD, J., ARCHIBALD, K.C.: Occurrence of so-called "myotonic discharges" in electromyography. Arch. Phys. Med. 39, 20-22 (1958).
125. GOODGOLD, J., EBERSTEIN, A.: An electromyographic study of induced myotonia in rats. Exp. Neurol. 21, 159-166 (1968).
126. GUTH, L.: "Trophic" influences of nerve on muscle. Physiol. Rev. 48, 645-687 (1968).
127. GUTH, L., SAMAHA, F.J.: Qualitative differences between actomyosin ATPase of slow and fast mammalian muscle. Exp. Neurol. 25, 138-152 (1970).
128. GUTH, L., SAMAHA, F.J., ALBERS, R.W.: The neural regulation of some phenotypic differences between the fiber types of mammalian skeletal muscle. Exp. Neurol. 26, 126-135 (1970).
129. GUTH, L., YELLIN, H.: The dynamic nature of the so-called "fiber types" of mammalian skeletal muscle. Exp. Neurol. 31, 277-300 (1971).
130. HALL-CRAGGS, E.C.B.: The longitudinal division of fibres in overloaded rat skeletal muscle. J. Anat. 107, 459-470 (1970).
131. HALL-CRAGGS, E.C.B., LAWRENCE, C.A.: Longitudinal fiber division in rat skeletal muscle. J. Physiol. (Lond.) 202, 76p (1969).
132. HARM, K.: Enzymaktivitätsbestimmungen in Leber und Muskel von Mäusen mit hereditärer Muskeldystrophie. Enzymol. Biol. Clin. 9, 205-218 (1968).
133. HARMAN, P.J., TASSONI, J.P., CURTIS, R.L., HOLLINSHEAD, M.B.: Muscular dystrophy in the mouse. In: Muscular dystrophy in man and animals (ed. G.H. BOURNE, M.L. GOLARZ), pp. 407-456. Basel: Karger 1963.
134. HARRIS, J.B.: The resting membrane potential of fibers of fast and slow twitch muscles in normal and dystrophic mice. J. Neurol. Sci. 12, 45-52 (1971).
135. HARRIS, J.B., WILSON, P.: Denervation in murine dystrophy. Nature 229, 61-62 (1971).
136. HASCHKE, R.H., HEILMEYER, L.M.G., Jr., MEYER, F., FISCHER, E.H.: Control of phosphorylase activity in a muscle glycogen particle. III. Regulation of phosphorylase phophatase. J. biol. Chem. 245, 6657-6663 (1970).

137. HASHIMOTO, T., KALUZA, J.S., BURSTONE, M.S.: The effect
of menadione and phenazine methosulfate on the tetrazolium
reduction system under histochemical conditions. J. Histochem. Cytochem. 12, 797-804 (1964).
138. HEENE, R.: Histochemischer Nachweis der Phosphorylasehemmung
durch 2,4-Dichlorphenoxyazetat (2,4-D) an Skelettmuskel und
Leber der Ratte. Naturwissenschaften 53, 308 (1966).
139. HEENE, R.: Hemmung glykogenbildender Enzyme durch 2,4-
Dichlorphenoxyazetat (2,4-D). Histochemie 8, 45-53 (1967).
140. HEENE, R.: Experimentell-histochemische Untersuchungen
zum Glykogenstoffwechsel des Skelettmuskels. Anat. Anz.
Erg.-Bd. 121, 45-48 (1968).
141. HEENE, R.: Histochemische und morphologische Befunde bei
experimenteller Myopathie durch 2,4-Dichlorphenoxyazetat
(2,4-D) beim Warmblüter. Acta neuropath. (Berlin) 10,
166-169 (1968).
142. HEENE, R.: Elektronenmikroskopische Befunde bei experimenteller Myopathie durch 2,4-Dichlorphenoxyazetat (2,4-D)
beim Warmblüter. Zur Entwicklung der Frühveränderungen bei
Myopathien. Dtsch. Z. Nervenheilk. 193, 265-278 (1968).
143. HEENE, R.: Fasertypen des Skelettmuskels. Nervenarzt 43,
323-326 (1972).
144. HEILMEYER, L.M.G., Jr., MEYER, F., HASCHKE, R.H., FISCHER,
E.H.: Control of phosphorylase activity in a muscle
glycogen particle. II. Activation by calcium. J. Biol.
Chem. 245, 6649-6656 (1970).
145. HEYCK, H., LAUDAHN, G.: Die progressiv-dystrophischen
Myopathien. Berlin, Heidelberg, New York: Springer 1969.
146. HICKS, S.P.: Brain metabolism in vivo. II. The distribution of lesions caused by azide, malononitrile, plasmocid
and dinitrophenol poisoning in rats. Arch. Path. (Chicago)
50, 545-561 (1950).
147. HILTON, S.M., JEFFRIES, M.G., VRBOVÁ, G.: Functional
specializations of the vascular bed of soleus. J. Physiol.
(Lond.) 206, 543-562 (1970).
148. HINTERBUCHNER, L.P., ANGYAN, A., HIRSCH, M.: Effect of
series of tetani on dystrophic and normal muscles of
mouse. Amer. J. Physiol. 211, 915-918 (1966).
149. HOLLIDAY, T.A., JULIAN, L.M., ASMUNDSON, V.S.: Muscle
growth in selected lines of muscular dystrophic chickens.
Anat. Rec. 160, 207-216 (1968).
150. HOLLIDAY, T.A., METER, J.R., van, JULIAN, L.M., ASMUNDSON,
V.S.: Electromyography of chickens with inherited muscular
dystrophy. Amer. J. Physiol. 209, 871-876 (1965).
151. HOLLOSZY, J.C.: Biochemical adaptations in muscle. Effects
of exercise on mitochondrial oxygen uptake and respiratory
enzyme activity in skeletal muscle. J. Biol. Chem. 242,
2278-2283 (1967).
153. HOOEY, M.A., JERRY, L.M.: The cardiomyopathy of muscular
dystrophy; report of two cases with a review of the
literature. Canad. Med. Ass. J. 90, 771 (1964).
154. HOOTON, B.T., WATTS, D.C.: Adenosine 5'-triphosphate-
creatine phosphotransferase from dystrophic mouse skeletal
muscle: A genetic lesion associated with the catalytic-
site thiol group. Biochem. J. 100, 637-646 (1966).
155. HORI, S.H.: Effect of EDTA on histochemical demonstration
of phosphorylase activity. J. Histochem. Cytochem. 14,
501-508 (1966).

156. HØSTMARK, A.T., HORN, R.S.: Stimulation of sensitivity of the glycogen phosphorylase-converting system in skeletal muscle by metabolic inhibitors. Biochim. Biophys. Acta 304, 389-396 (1973).

157. HUDGSON, P., PEARCE, G.W., WALTON, J.N.: Pre-clinical muscular dystrophy: histopathological changes observed on muscle biopsy. Brain 90, 565-576 (1967).

158. HULS, H.N., LEONARD, S.L.: Phosphorylase activity in denervated skeletal muscle. Proc. Soc. exp. Biol. Med. (N.Y.) 108, 224-228 (1961).

159. IONASESCU, V., VUIA, O., LUCA, N., POPA, P., ANUTEI, V., ANUTEI, E.: Biochemical and histopathological studies of the carrier state in Duchenne's muscular dystrophy. Confin. Neurol. 30, 289-300 (1969).

160. JACOBS, H., OKABE, K., YUE, R., KEUTEL, H., ZITER, F., PALMIERI, R., TYLER, F., KUBY, S.A.: A comparison of normal human ATP-creatine transphosphorylases with those from progressive muscular dystrophy tissues. Fed. Proc. Fed. Amer. Soc. exp. Biol. 28, 346 (495 P)(1969).

161. JAMES, T.W.: Observations on the cardiovascular involvement, including the cardiac conduction system, in progressive muscular dystrophy. Amer. Heart J. 63, 48-56 (1962).

162. JASMIN, G.: Histochemical studies on denervation, chemically induced and hereditary forms of myopathies. Ann. N.Y. Acad. Sci. 138, 186-198 (1966).

163. JASMIN, G.: Hyperbasophilia of muscle fibers in healthy siblings of a dystrophic Syrian hamster line. In: Muscle Diseases. Proc. of an intern. Congr., Milan 19-21 May 1969 (ed. J.N. WALTON, N. CANAL, G. SCARLATO), pp. 53-55. Amsterdam: Excerpta Medica 1970.

164. JASMIN, G., BAJUSZ, E.: Myocardial lesions in strain 129 dystrophic mice. Nature 193, 181 (1962).

165. JEDRZEJOWSKA, H., JOHNSON, A.G., WOOLF, A.L.: The intramuscular nerve endings in muscular dystrophy. A biopsy study. Acta Neuropath. (Berlin) 5, 225-242 (1965).

166. JENKINS, K., HIDIROGLOU, M., MACAY, R.R., PROULX, J.R.: Influence of selenium and linoleic acid on the development of nutritional muscular dystrophy in beef calves, lambs and rabbits. Can. J. Anim. Sci. 50, 137-146 (1970).

167. JERUSALEM, F., ENGEL, A.G., GOMEZ, M.R.: Duchenne Dystrophy - II. Morphometric study of motor end-plate fine structure. Brain 97, 123-130 (1974).

168. JOHNSON, M., PEARSE, A.G.E.: Differentiation of fibre types in normal and dystrophic hamster muscle. J. Neurol. Sci. 12, 459-472 (1971).

169. JULIAN, L.M., ASMUNDSON, V.S.: Muscular dystrophy of the chicken. In: Muscular Dystrophy in Man and Animals (ed. G.H. BOURNE, M.N. GOLARZ), pp. 457-498. Basel: Karger 1963.

170. KAKULAS, B.A.: Myopathy affecting the Rottnest quokka (Setonix brachyurus) reversed by α-tocopherol. Nature 191, 402-403 (1961).

171. KAKULAS, B.A., ADAMS, R.D.: Principles of myopathology as illustrated in the nutritional myopathy of the Rottnest quokka (Setonix brachyurus). Ann. N.Y. Acad. Sci. 138, 90-101 (1966).

172. KANDUTSCH, A.A., RUSSELL, A.E.: Creatine and creatinine in tissues and urine of mice with hereditary muscular dystrophy. Amer. J. Physiol. 194, 553-556 (1958).
173. KAPLAN, N.O., CAHN, R.D.: Lactic dehydrogenases and muscular dystrophy in the chicken. Proc. Nat. Acad. Sci. (Wash.) 48, 2123-2130 (1962).
174. KARPATI, G., ENGEL, W.K.: Histochemical investigation of fiber type ratios with the myofibrillar ATPase reaction in normal and denervated skeletal muscles of guinea pig. Amer. J. Anat. 122, 145-156 (1968).
175. KERPOLLA, W.: Inhibition of phosphorylase with cortisone and its activation with adrenaline in the rabbit. Endocrinology 51, 192-202 (1952).
176. KEY, J.L.: Ribonucleic acid and protein synthesis as essential processes for cell elongation. Plant Physiol. 39, 365-370 (1964).
177. KLEINE, T.O.: Evidence for the release of enzyme from different organs in Duchenne's muscular dystrophy. Clin. chim. Acta 29, 227-232 (1970).
178. KLEINE, T.O., CHLOND, R.: Zur enzymatischen Differentialdiagnose der Organbeteiligung bei der progressiven Muskeldystrophie (Erb) während dreier Therapieversuche. Enzymol. Biol. Clin. 10, 39-67 (1969).
179. KOWALSKI, K., GORDON, E.E., MARTINEZ, A., ADAMEK, J.: Changes in enzyme activities of various muscle fiber types in rat induced by different exercises. J. Histochem. Cytochem. 17, 601-607 (1969).
180. KREBS, G.E., LANGE, R.J., de, KEMP, R.G., RILEY, W.D.: Activation of skeletal muscle phosphorylase. Pharmacol. Rev. 18, 163-171 (1966).
181. KUGELBERG, E., EDSTRÖM, L.: Differential histochemical effects of muscle contractions on phosphorylase and glycogen in various types of fibers: relation to fatigue. J. Neurol. Neurosurg. Psychiat. 31, 415-423 (1968).
182. KUHN, E., STEIN, W.: Modell-Myotonie nach 2,4-Dichlorphenoxyazetat bei der Ratte. Bestimmung des Glucose-6-Phosphates, Adenosin-triphosphates und ADP im Musculus pectoralis. Klin. Wschr. 42, 1215-1216 (1964).
183. KUHN, E., STEIN, W.: Modellmyotonie nach 2,4-Dichlorphenoxyazetat (2,4-D) bei der Ratte. In vitro- und in vivo-Untersuchungen über den Einfluß von 2,4-D auf den Energiestoffwechsel des Muskels. Klin. Wschr. 43, 673-677 (1965).
184. KUHN, E., STEIN, W.: Modellmytonie nach 2,4-Dichlorphenoxyazetat (2,4-D). Calciumaufnahme der Vesikel des sarkoplasmatischen Reticulums unter 2,4-D. Klin. Wschr. 44, 700-702 (1966).
185. KUNZE, K.: Das Sauerstoffdruckfeld im normalen und pathologisch veränderten Muskel. Schriftenreihe Neurologie, Bd. 3. Berlin, Heidelberg, New York: Springer 1969.
186. LARSEN, M., COUCH, J.R., ENZMANN, F., BOLER, L., MUSTAFA, H.T., FOLKERS, K.: Vitamin activity of coenzyme Q in chickens and turkeys. Int. Z. Vitaminforsch. 39, 447-456 (1969).
187. LEHOCZKY, T., SÓS, J., HALASY, M.: Animal experiments on the aetiology of myelopathy. Akadémiai Kiadó Budapest, 1964, pp. 198-203.

188. LENMAN, J.A.R.: Effect of denervation on the resting
     membrane potential of healthy and dystrophic muscle.
     J. Neurol. Neurosurg. Psychiat. $\underline{28}$, 525-528 (1965).
189. LEONARD, S.L.: Phosphorylase and glycogen levels in
     skeletal muscles of mice with hereditary myopathy.
     Proc. Soc. exp. Biol. Med. (N.Y.) $\underline{96}$, 720-722 (1957).
190. LEONARD, S.L.: Phosphorylase activity in normal and ab-
     normal muscle. In: Exploratory Concepts in Muscular
     Dystrophy and Related Disorders (ed. A.T. MILHORAT).
     Amsterdam: Excerpta Medica, Int. Congr. Ser. 147 (1967).
191. LIPSCHUTZ, M.D.: Les voies atteintes chez les jeunes
     rats manquant de vitamine E. Rev. Neurol. $\underline{65}$, 221-233
     (1936).
192. MACDONALD, R.D., ENGEL, A.G.: Experimental chloroquine
     myopathy. J. Neuropath. exp. Neurol. $\underline{29}$, 479-499 (1970).
193. MANN, O., DELEON, A.C., Jr., PERLOFF, J.K., SIMANIS, J.,
     HORRIGAN, F.D.: Duchenne's muscular dystrophy. The
     electrocardiogram in female relatives. Amer. J. Med.
     Sci. $\underline{255}$, 376-381 (1968).
194. MASON, K.E.: Effect of nutritional deficiencies upon
     muscle. In: Structure and Function of Muscle, Vol. III
     (ed. G.H. BOURNE), pp. 171-207. New York: Academic Press
     1960.
195. MASON, K.E., DJU, M.Y., CHAPIN, S.J.: Vitamin-E-content
     of tissues in progressive muscular dystrophy. Proc. 1st
     and 2nd Med. Confer. Musc. Dystr. Assns. Amer. 1951-1952,
     p. 94.
196. MASON, K.E., EMMEL, A.F.: Vitamin E and muscle pigment
     in rat. Anat. Rec. $\underline{92}$, 33-59 (1945).
197. MATHISEN, J.S., MELLGREN, S.I.: Some observations con-
     cerning the role of phenazine methosulfate in histo-
     chemical dehydrogenase methods. J. Histochem. Cytochem.
     $\underline{13}$, 408-409 (1965).
198. MCCAMAN, M.W.: Dehydrogenase activities in dystrophic
     mice. Science $\underline{132}$, 621-622 (1960).
199. MCCAMAN, M.W.: Enzyme studies of skeletal muscle in mice
     with hereditary muscular dystrophy. Amer. J. Physiol. $\underline{205}$,
     897-901 (1963).
200. MCCOMAS, A.J., MOSSAWY, S.J.: Excitability of muscle
     fiber membranes in dystrophic mice. J. Neurol. Neurosurg.
     Psychiat. $\underline{29}$, 440-445 (1966).
201. MCCOMAS, A.J., THOMAS, H.C.: A study of the muscle twitch
     in the Duchenne type muscular dystrophy. J. Neurol. Sci. $\underline{7}$,
     309-312 (1968).
202. MCCOMAS, A.J., SICA, R.E.P., CURRIE, S.: Muscular dystrophy:
     Evidence for a neural factor. Nature $\underline{226}$, 1263-1264 (1970).
203. MCCOMAS, A.J., SICA, R.E.P., CURRIE, S.: An electro-
     physiological study of Duchenne dystrophy. J. Neurol.
     Neurosurg. Psychiat. $\underline{34}$, 461-468 (1971).
204. MCINTYRE, A.R., BENNETT, A.L., BRODKEY, J.S.: Muscle
     dystrophy in mice of the Bar Harbor strain. A.M.A. Arch.
     Neurol. Psychiat. $\underline{81}$, 678-683 (1959).
205. MEIER, H.: Histochemical observations in preclinical
     mouse muscular dystrophy. Amer. J. Path. $\underline{50}$, 691-706
     (1967).
206. MEIER, H., HOAG, W.T., HOAG, W.G.: Preclinical histo-
     pathology of mouse muscular dystrophy. Arch. Path. $\underline{80}$,
     165-170 (1965).

207. MEIJER, A.E.F.H.: Improved histochemical method for the demonstration of the activity of α-glucan phosphorylase. I. The use of glucosyl acceptor dextran. Histochemie 12, 244-252 (1968).

208. MEIJER, A.E.F.H.: Improved histochemical method for the demonstration of the activity of α-glucan phosphorylase. II. Relation of molecular weight of glucosyl acceptor dextran to activation of phosphorylase. Histochemie 16, 134-143 (1968).

209. MEYER, F., HEILMEYER, L.M.G., Jr., HASCHKE, R.H., FISCHER, E.H.: Control of phosphorylase activity in a muscle glycogen particle. I. Isolation and characterization of the protein-glycogen complex. J. biol. Chem. 245, 6642-6648 (1970).

210. MICHELSON, A.M., RUSSELL, E.S., HARMAN, P.J.: Dystrophia muscularis: a hereditary primary myopathy in the house mouse. Proc. Nat. Acad. Sci. U.S. 41, 1079-1984 (1955).

211. MILHORAT, A.T., SHAFIQ, S.A., GOLDSTONE, L.: Changes in muscle structure in dystrophic patients, carriers and normal siblings seen by electron microscopy; correlation with levels of serum creatinephosphokinase (CPK). Ann. N.Y. Acàd. Sci. 138, 246-292 (1966).

212. MOMMAERTS, W.F.H.M.: The energetics of muscular contraction. Physiol. Rev. 49, 427-502 (1969).

213. MONCKTON, G., NIHEI, T.: The localization of increased protein synthesis in mouse muscular dystrophy. In: Basic Research in Myology (ed. B.A. KAKULAS), Part 1, pp. 271-280. Amsterdam: Excerpta Medica; New York: American Elsevier 1973.

214. MONCKTON, G., MARUSYK, H.: Autoradiographic studies in heart muscle of the normal and dystrophic mouse. Abstr. IIIrd Internat. Congr. Muscle Dis., Newcastle-upon-Tyne, England, Sept. 15-21, 1974. Amsterdam: Excerpta Medica 334, 44 1974.

215. MONRO, P.: Early biochemical changes in plasmocid myopathy. J. Neurol. Neurosurg. Psychiat. 31, 633-640 (1968).

216. NADKARNI, B.B., HUNT, B., HEGGTVEIT, H.A.: Early ultrastructural and biochemical changes in the myopathic hamster heart. Abstr. 3rd Annual Meeting of the Internat. Study Group for Research in Cardiac Metabolism, Stowe, Vt., 1970.

217. NEELY, W.B., BALL, C.D., HAMNER, C.L., SELL, H.M.: Effects of 2,4-Dichlorphenoxyacetic acid on the invertase, phosphorylase and pectin methoxylase activity in the stems and leaves of the red kidney bean plants. Plant. Physiol. 25, 525-528 (1950).

218. NEGRI, S., PACINI, L.: Considerazioni elettromiografiche sulla distrofia muscolare pseudo-hipertrofica di Duchenne. Riv. Neurobiol. 5, 525-560 (1959).

219. NELSON, A.A., FITZHUGH, O.G.: Chloroquine; pathologic changes observed in rats which for 2 years had been fed various proportions. Arch. Path. 45, 454-462 (1948).

220. NESHEIM, M.C., LEONARD, S.L., SCOTT, M.L.: Alterations in some biochemical constituents of skeletal muscle of vitamin-E deficient chicks. J. Nutr. 68, 359-369 (1959).

221. NOTHACKER, W.G., NETSKY, M.G.: Myocardial lesions in progressive muscular dystrophy. Arch. Path. 50, 578-590 (1950).

84

222. OFTEDAL, S.-I., MUNTHE-KAAS, A.W.: Chloroquine neuro-
     myopathy. Acta Neurol. Scand. 43, Suppl. 31, 147-148
     (1967). (Proc. 18th Congr. Scand. Neurol., Helsinki 1967).
223. OLCOTT, H.S.: Paralysis in young of vitamin-E deficient
     female rats. J. Nutrition 15, 221-227 (1938).
224. ONISHI, S., BAJUSZ, E., BÜCHNER, F., RICKERS, K.: Herz-
     muskelhypertrophie bei erbbedingter Myopathie des syrischen
     Hamsters nach elektronenmikroskopischen Untersuchungen.
     Beitr. Path. Anat. 140, 119-141 (1970).
225. PADYKULA, H., GAUTHIER, G.F.: Ultrastructural features
     of three fiber types in the rat diaphragm. Anat. Rec. 157,
     296-297 (1967).
226. PADYKULA, H., HERMAN, E.: The specifity of the histo-
     chemical method for ATPase. J. Histochem. Cytochem. 3,
     170-195 (1955).
227. PAPPENHEIMER, A.M.: Certain nutritional disorders of
     laboratory animals due to vitamin-E deficiency. J. Mt.
     Sinai Hosp. 7, 65-76 (1940).
228. PAPPENHEIMER, A.M., GOETTSCH, M.: Effect of nerve section
     upon development of nutritional muscular dystrophy in
     young rats. Proc. Soc. exp. Biol. Med. 43, 313-316 (1940).
229. PEARCE, G.W.: Electron microscopy in the study of muscular
     dystrophy. In: Muscular Dystrophy in Man and Animals (ed.
     G.H. BROUNE, M.N. GOLARZ). Basel: Karger 1963.
230. PEARCE, G.W.: Electron microscopy in the study of muscular
     dystrophy. Ann. N.Y. Acad. Sci. 138, 138-150 (1966).
231. PEARCE, G.W., WALTON, J.N.: Progressive muscular dystrophy:
     the histopathological changes in skeletal muscle obtained
     by biopsy. J. Path. Bact. 83, 535-550 (1962).
232. PEARCE, G.W., WALTON, J.N.: A histological study of muscle
     from the Bar Harbor strain of dystrophic mice. J. Path.
     Bact. 86, 25-33 (1963).
233. PEARSE, A.G.E.: Histochemistry, Vol. I, 3rd edn., London:
     J. and A. Churchill 1968. Vol. II, 3rd edn., 1972.
234. PEARSON, C.M.: Pathology of human muscular dystrophy.
     In: Muscular Dystrophy in Man and Animals (ed. G.H. BOURNE,
     N.M. GOLARZ). Basel: Karger 1963.
235. PERLOFF, J.K., ROBERTS, W.C., DELEON, A.C., O'DOHERTY, D.:
     The distinctive electrocardiogram of Duchenne's progressive
     muscular dystrophy. An electrocardiographic-pathologic
     correlative study. Amer. J. Med. 42, 179-188 (1967).
236. PETER, J.B.: Changes with age in shuttle enzymes of white
     and red muscle from normal and dystrophic chickens. In:
     Exploratory Concepts in Muscular Dystrophy and Related
     Disorders (ed. A.T. MILHORAT). Int. Congr. Ser. No. 147,
     pp. 327-338. Amsterdam: Excerpta Medica 1967.
237. PETER, J.B., VERHAAG, D.A., WORSFOLD, M.: Studies of
     steroid myopathy. Examination of the effect of triamcino-
     lone on mitochondria and sarcotubular vesicles of rat
     skeletal muscle. Biochem. Pharmacol. 19, 1627-1636 (1970).
238. PETERS, R.F., RICHARDSON, M.C., SMALL, M., WHITE, A.M.:
     Some biochemical effects of triamcinolone acetonide on
     rat liver and muscle. Biochem. J. 116, 349-355 (1970).
239. PETTE, D., BRANDAU, H.: Enzymhistiogramme und Enzym-
     Aktivitätsmuster der Rattenleber. Enzym. Biol. Clin.
     (Basel) 6, 79-122 (1966).

240. PFEIFFER, C.: Elektronenmikroskopische Untersuchungen am Mäusestamm 129 mit hereditärer Muskeldystrophie. Arch. orthop. Unfall-Chir. 54, 425-442 (1962).

241. PLATZER, A.C., CHASE, W.H.: Histologic alterations in preclinical mouse muscular dystrophy. Amer. J. Path. 44, 931-946 (1964).

242. PREISS, D., HAAG, D., GOERTTLER, K.: Beeinflussung der DNS-Reduplikation kultivierter embryonaler Skelettmuskelzellen durch das Herbicid 2,4-Dichlorphenoxyessigsäure. Naturwissenschaften 59, 173 (1972).

243. PRICE, H.M., PEASE, D.C., PEARSON, C.M.: Selective actin filament and Z band degeneration induced by plasmocid, an electron microscopic study. Lab. Invest. 11, 549-562 (1962).

244. RENIERS, J., MARTIN, L., JORIS, C.: Histochemical and quantitative analysis of muscle biopsies. J. Neurol. Sci. 10, 349-367 (1970).

245. REZNIK, M., HANSEN, J.L.: Mitochondria in degenerating and regenerating skeletal muscle. Arch. Path. 87, 601-608 (1969).

246. RINGSTED, A.: Preliminary note on appearance of paresis in adult rats suffering from chronic avitaminosis E. Biochem. J. 29, 788-795 (1935).

247. ROMANUL, F.C.A.: Enzymes in muscle. I. Histochemical studies of enzymes in individual muscle fibers. Arch. Neurol. (Chicago) 11, 355-368 (1964).

248. ROMANUL, F.C.A.: Capillary supply and metabolism of muscle fibers. Arch. Neurol. 12, 497-509 (1965).

249. RONZONI, E., BERG, L., LANDAU, W.: Enzyme studies in progressive muscular dystrophy. Res. Publ. Ass. nerv. ment. Dis. 38, 721-729 (1960).

250. ROSS, M.H., PAPPAS, G.D., HARMAN, P.J.: Alterations in muscle fine structure in hereditary muscular dystrophy of mice. Lab. Invest. 9, 388-403 (1960).

251. ROVETTA, P., SALA, E.: Attività da inserzione di tipo miotonico registrata in casa di distrofia muscolare progressiva. Riv. Neurol. 29, 178-187 (1959).

252. ROWE, R.W.D., GOLDSPINK, G.: Muscle fiber growth in five different muscles in both sexes of mice. I. Normal mice. J. Anat. 104, 519-530 (1969).

253. ROWE, R.W.D., GOLDSPINK, G.: Muscle fiber growth in five different muscles in both sexes of mice. II. Dystrophic mice. J. Anat. 104, 531-538 (1969).

254. ROWAN, K.S.: Phosphorus metabolism in plants. In: Internat. Rev. Cytol. (ed. G.H. BOURNE, J.F. DANIELLI), Vol. 19, p. 301-390. New York, London: Academic Press 1966.

255. ROY, A., DUBOWITZ, V.: Carrier detection in Duchenne muscular dystrophy. A comparative study of electron microscopy, light microscopy and serum enzymes. J. Neurol. Sci. 11, 65-80 (1970).

256. ROY, B.P., LAWS, J.F., THOMSON, A.R.: Preparation and properties of creatine kinase from the breast muscle of normal and dystrophic chicken (Gallus domesticus). Biochem. J. 120, 177-185 (1970).

257. RULON, R.R., SCHOTTELIUS, D.D., SCHOTTELIUS, B.A.: Phosphorylase activation in stimulated dystrophic mouse muscle. Amer. J. Physiol. 202, 821-823 (1962).

258. RUMERY, R.E., HAMPTON, J.C.: Microscopic and submicroscopic observations on skeletal muscle from vitamin-E deficient rats. Anat. Rec. 133, 1-11 (1959).

259. SAMAHA, F.J., GUTH, Ll., ALBERS, R.W.: Phenotypic differences between the actomyosin ATPase of the three fiber types of mammalian skeletal muscle. Exp. Neurol. 26, 120-125 (1970).

260. SANDOW, A., BRUST, M.: Contractility of dystrophic mouse muscles. Amer. J. Physiol. 194, 557-563 (1958).

261. SCHAPIRA, G., DREYFUS, J.C., SCHAPIRA, F., KRUH, J.: Glycogenolytic enzymes in human progressive muscular dystrophy. Amer. J. Phys. Med. 34, 313-319 (1955).

262. SCHMALBRUCH, H.: Die quergestreiften Muskelfasern des Menschen. Erg. Anat. Entwicklungsgesch. (edit. A. BRODAL, H. HILD, R. ORTMANN et al.) 43, 1, Berlin, Heidelberg, New York: Springer 1970.

263. SCHOLLER, J., JONES, D., LITTARU, G.P., FOLKERS, K.: Therapy of hereditary mouse muscular dystrophy with coenzyme Q7. Biochem. Biophys. Res. Commun. 41, 1298-1305 (1970).

264. SCHOTLAND, D.L.: An electron microscopic study of target fibers, targetlike fibers and related abnormalities in human muscle. J. Neuropath. exp. Neurol. 28, 214-228 (1969).

265. SCHRÖDER, J.M., KUHN, E.: Zur Ultrastruktur der Muskelfaser bei der experimentellen "Myotonie" mit 20,25-Diazacholesterin. Virchows Arch. Abt. A, Path. Anat. 344, 181-195 (1968).

266. SCOTT, M.L.: Studies on the interrelationship of selenium, vitamin E, and sulfur amino acids in a nutritional myopathy of the chick. Ann. N.Y. Acad. Sci. 138, 82-89 (1966).

267. SEILER, D., FIEHN, W., KUHN, E.: Disturbances in Cholesterol Biosynthesis as a Cause of Experimental Myotonia. Abstr. IIIrd Internat. Congr. Muscle Dis., Newcastle-upon-Tyne, England Sept. 15-21, 1974. Amsterdam: Excerpta Medica 334, 148 1974.

268. SENGES, J., RÜDEL, R.: Experimental myotonia in mammalian skeletal muscle: changes in contractile properties. Pflügers Arch. 331, 315-323 (1972).

269. SHAFIQ, S.A., GORYCKI, M.A., MILHORAT, A.T.: An electron microscope study of fibre types in normal and dystrophic muscles of the mouse. J. Anat. 104, 281-294 (1969).

270. SHANK, R.E., GILDER, H., HOAGLAND, C.L.: Studies on diseases of muscle. I. Progressive muscular dystrophy; a clinical review of 40 cases. Arch. Neurol. (Chicago) 52, 431-442 (1944).

271. SIGEL, P., PETTE, D.: Intracellular localization of glycogenolytic and glycolytic enzymes in white and red rabbit skeletal muscle. J. Histochem. Cytochem. 17, 225-237 (1969).

272. SICA, R.E.P., MCCOMAS, A.J.: An electrophysiological investigation of limb-girdle and facioscapulohumeral dystrophy. J. Neurol. Neurosurg. Psychiat. 34, 469-474 (1971).

273. SIMON, E.J., GROSS, C.S., LESSEL, I.M.: Turnover of muscle and liver proteins in mice with hereditary muscular dystrophy. Arch. Biochem. Biophys. 96, 41-46 (1962).

274. SLUCKA, C.: The electrocardiogram in Duchenne progressive muscular dystrophy. Circulation 38, 933-940 (1968).
275. SMITH, B.: Histological and histochemical changes in the muscles of rabbits given the corticosteroid triamcinolone. Neurology (Minneap.) 14, 857-863 (1964).
276. SMITH, B.: Histochemical changes in muscle necrosis and regeneration. J. Path. Bact. 89, 139-143 (1965).
277. SMITH, B., O'GRADY, F.: Experimental chloroquine myopathy. J. Neurol. Neurosurg. Psychiat. 29, 255-258 (1966).
278. SOMERS, J.E., WINER, N.: Reversible myopathy and myotonia following administration of a hypocholesterolemic agent. Neurology (Minneap.) 16, 761-765 (1966).
279. SORDAHL, L.A., CROW, C.A., KRAFT, G.H., SCHWARTZ, A.: Some ultrastructural and biochemical aspects of heart mitochondria associated with development: fetal and cardio-myopathic tissue. J. Mol. Cell Cardiol. 4, 1-10 (1972).
280. STAMP, W.G., LESKER, P.A.: Enzyme studies related to sex differences in mice with hereditary muscular dystrophy. Amer. J. Physiol. 213, 587-591 (1967).
281. STEIN, J.M., PADYKULA, H.A.: Histochemical classification of individual skeletal muscle fibers of the rat. Amer. J. Anat. 110, 103-124 (1962).
282. STEIN, W., KUHN, E.: Modellmyotonie nach 2,4-Dichlor-phenoxyazetat (2,4-D). Isoliertes Rattenzwerchfell als einfaches Untersuchungsobjekt. Klin. Wschr. 46, 328-330 (1968).
283. STORSTEIN, O.: The heart in progressive muscular dystrophy. Exp. Med. Surg. 22, 13-23 (1964).
284. STORSTEIN, O., KLINGE, F.O.: Heart involvement in progressive muscular dystrophy. Acta Psychiat. Scand. 36, 489-496 (1961).
285. SUGITA, H., TYLER, F.H.: Pathogenesis of muscular dystrophy. Trans. Ass. Amer. Physns. 76, 231 (1963).
286. SUSHEELA, A.K., HUDGSON, P., WALTON, J.N.: Murine muscular dystrophy. Some histochemical and biochemical observations. J. Neurol. Sci. 7, 437-463 (1968).
287. SUSHEELA, A.K., HUDGSON, P., WALTON, J.N.: Histological and histochemical studies of experimentally-induced degeneration and regeneration in normal and dystrophic mouse muscle. J. Neurol. Sci. 9, 423-442 (1969).
288. SUSHEELA, A.K., WALTON, J.N.: Note on the distribution of histochemical fiber types in some normal human muscles. A study on autopsy material. J. Neurol. Sci. 8, 201-207 (1969).
289. SWANSON, M.A.: Studies on the structure of polysaccharides. IV. Relation of the iodine color to the structure. J. Biol. Chem. 172, 825-837 (1948).
290. TAKASU, T., HUGHES, B.P.: Lactate dehydrogenase isozyme patterns in human skeletal muscle. I. Variation of isozyme pattern in the adult. J. Neurol. Neurosurg. Psychiat. 32, 175-180 (1969).
291. TAKEUCHI, T.: Histochemical demonstration of branching enzyme (Amylo-1,4 →1,6-transglucosidase) in animal tissues. J. Histochem. Cytochem. 6, 208-216 (1958).
292. TAKEUCHI, T., GLENNER, G.G.: Histochemical demonstration of a pathway for polysaccharide synthesis from uridine di-phosphoglucose. J. Histochem. Cytochem. 8, 227-230 (1960).

293. TAKEUCHI, T., KURIAKI, H.: Histochemical detection of
phosphorylase in animal tissue. J. Histochem. Cytochem.
3, 153-160 (1955).
294. TASSONI, J.P., MANTEL, L., HARMAN, P.J.: Enzyme alterations in muscle cells from mice with hereditary dystrophy.
Exp. Cell Res. 35, 219-229 (1964).
295. TICE, L.W., ENGEL, A.G.: Effects of glucocorticoids on
fine structure of red and white rat muscle. J. Cell Biol.
27, 106A-107A (1965).
296. TICE, L.W., ENGEL, A.G.: The effects of glucocorticoids
on red and white muscles of the rat. Amer. J. Path. 50,
311-333 (1967).
297. TUREEN, L.L., SIMONS, R.: Enzyme changes within muscle
fibers in genetic and nutritional muscular dystrophy.
Proc. Soc. exp. Biol. Med. 129, 384-390 (1968).
298. VAN BREEMEN, V.L.: Ultrastructure of human muscle.
II. Observations on dystrophic striated muscle fibers.
Amer. J. Path. 37, 337-341 (1960).
299. VAN VLEET, J.F., HALL, B.V., SIMON, J.S.: Vitamin E
deficiency: a sequential light and electron microscopic
study of skeletal muscle degeneration in weanling rabbits.
Amer. J. Path. 52, 1067-1080 (1968).
300. VAN WIJE, M., BLANCHAER, M.C., JACYK, W.R.: The oxidation
of lactate and α-glycerophosphate by red and white skeletal
muscle: II. Histochemical studies. J. Histochem. Cytochem.
11, 505-510 (1963).
301. VIGNOS, P.J.: Experimental corticosteroid myopathy. A
correlated histochemical and biochemical study. In: Advances in Neuromuscular Diseases (ed. G. SERRATRICE), p.
549. Paris: L'expansion scientifique française 1971.
302. VIGNOS, P.J., GREENE, R.: Oxidative respiration of skeletal
muscle in experimental corticosteroid myopathy. J. Lab.
clin. Med. 81, 365-378 (1973).
303. WACHSTEIN, M., MEISEL, E.: Succinic dehydrogenase activity in myocardial infarction and in induced myocardial
necrosis. Amer. J. Path. 31, 353-366 (1955).
304. WALTON, J.N., GARDNER-MEDWIN, D., HUDGSON, P.: Carrier
detection in the Duchenne type muscular dystrophy. Int.
Congr. Ser. 154, p. 14. Amsterdam: Excerpta Medica 1967.
305. WALTON, J.N., NATRASS, F.J.: On the classification, natural
history and treatment of the myopathies. Brain 77, 169-231
(1954).
306. WALTON, J.N., PENNINGTON, R.J.T.: Studies on human muscular
dystrophy with particular reference to methods of carrier
detection. Ann. N.Y. Acad. Sci. 138, 315-328 (1966).
307. WECHSLER, W.: Comparative electron microscopic studies
on various forms of muscle atrophies and dystrophies in
animals and man. Ann. N.Y. Acad. Sci. 138, 113-137 (1966).
308. WECHSLER, W., PABELICK, W.: Erbliche Muskeldystrophien
beim Tier. In: Progressive Muskeldystrophie, Myotonie,
Myasthenie (edit. E. KUHN), pp. 165-177. Berlin, Heidelberg,
New York: Springer 1966.
309. WEINSTOCK, J.M., EPSTEIN, S., MILHORAT, A.T.: Enzyme
studies in muscular dystrophy. III. In: Hereditary muscle
dystrophy in mice. Proc. Soc. exp. Biol. Med. 99, 272-276
(1958).

310. WELSH, J.D., LYNN, T.N., HAASE, G.R.: Cardiac findings
     in 73 patients with muscular dystrophy. Arch. Intern.
     Med. 112, 199-206 (1963).
311. WEST, W.T.: Muscular dystrophy of vitamin-E deficiency.
     In: Muscular dystrophy in man and animals (ed. G.H. BOURNE,
     M.N. GOLARZ). Basel: Karger 1963.
312. WEST, W.T., MEIER, H., HOAG, W.G.: Hereditary mouse mus-
     cular dystrophy with particular emphasis on pathogenesis
     and attempts at therapy. Ann. N.Y. Acad. Sci. 138, 1-13
     (1966).
313. WINER, N., KLACHKO, D.M., BURNS, T.W., BAER, R.D.:
     Electromyographic myotonic response induced by cholesterol-
     lowering agents. Arch. Phys. Med. 46, 499 (1965).
314. WINER, N., KLACHKO, D.M., BAER, R.D., LANGLEY, P.L., BURNS,
     Th.W.: Myotonic response induced by inhibitors of cholesterol
     biosynthesis. Science 153, 312-313 (1966).
315. WOLF, A., PAPPENHEIMER, A.M.: Central nervous system in
     vitamin-E deficient rats. Arch. Neurol. Psychiat. 48,
     538-551 (1942).
316. YELLIN, H., GUTH, L.: The histochemical classification
     of muscle fibers. Exp. Neurol. 26, 424-432 (1970).
317. YOUNG, H.L., YOUNG, W., EDELMAN, I.S.: Electrolyte and
     liquid composition of skeletal and·cardiac muscle in mice
     with hereditary muscle dystrophy. Amer. J. Physiol. 197,
     487-490 (1959).
318. ZALKIN, H., TAPPEL, A.L., CALDWELL, K.A., SHIBKO, S.,
     DESAI, I.D., HOLLIDAY, T.A.: Increased lysosomal enzymes
     in muscular dystrophy of vitamin-E deficient rabbits.
     J. Biol. Chem. 237, 2678-2682 (1962).
319. ZELLWEGER, H., DURNIN, R., SIMPSON, J.: The diagnostic
     significance of serum enzymes and electrocardiogram in
     various muscular dystrophies. Acta Neurol. Scand. 48,
     87-101 (1972).

Subject Index

Abbreviations: CMD = chicken muscular dystrophy
                CMH = cardiomyopathy of Syrian hamster
                HMD = hamster muscular dystrophy
                MMD = mouse muscular dystrophy
                PMD = progressive muscular dystrophy of man

Schriftenreihe Neurologie – Neurology Series

Herausgeber: H. J. BAUER, H. GÄNSHIRT, P. VOGEL.

Die Bezieher des „Archiv für Psychiatrie und Nervenkrankheiten", des „Journal of Neurology / Zeitschrift für Neurologie" und des „Zentralblatt für die gesamte Neurologie und Psychiatrie" erhalten die Schriftenreihe zu einem um 10% ermäßigten Vorzugspreis. Preisänderungen vorbehalten.

F. Láhoda, A. Ross, W. Issel
EMG Primer
A Guide to Practical Electromyography
and Electroneurography. With a
Preface by A. Schrader. English Version
by J. Payan
30 figs. X, 60 pages. 1974
DM 28,–; US $12.10

D. Barker, C.C. Hunt, A.K. McIntyre
Muscle Receptors
Editor: C.C. Hunt
128 figs. VIII, 310 pages. 1974
(Handbook of Sensory Physiology,
Vol. 3, Part 2)
Cloth DM 130,–; US $55.90

Prices are subject to change without
notice

Journals

Acta Neurochirurgica
Official Organ of the European
Association of Neurosurgical Societies
(Springer-Verlag, Wien · New York)

Acta Neuropathologica
Organ of the Research Group for
Neuropathology, of the Research
Group for Comparative Neuropathology,
and of the Research Group for Neuro-
oncology of the World Federation of
Neurology

Experimental Brain Research

Journal of Neural Transmission
Formerly "Journal of Neuro-Visceral
Relations". Journal of the International
Society for Neurovegetative Research
Founded in 1950 as "Acta Neuro-
vegetativa" by Carmen Coronini and
Alexander Sturm
(Springer-Verlag, Wien · New York)

Journal of Neurology Zeitschrift für Neurologie
Organ der Deutschen Gesellschaft für
Neurologie und der Deutschen
Gesellschaft für Neurochirurgie

Neuroradiology
Organ of the European Society of
Neuroradiology

Sample copies as well as subscription
and back-volume information available
upon request

Please address:

Springer-Verlag
Werbeabteilung 4021
D 1000 Berlin 33
Heidelberger Platz 3

or

Springer-Verlag
New York Inc.
Promotion Department
175 Fifth Avenue
New York, N.Y. 10010

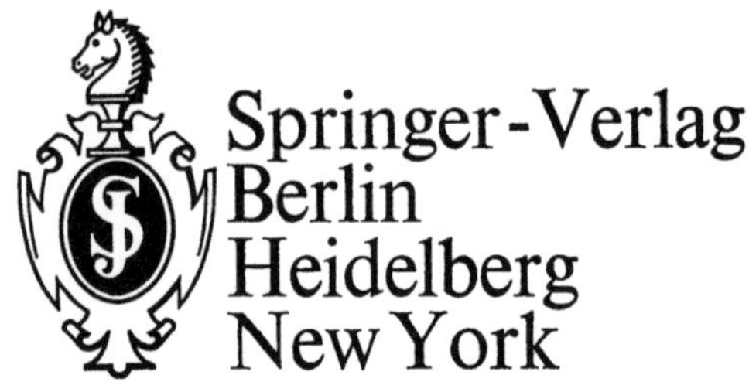

Springer-Verlag
Berlin
Heidelberg
New York